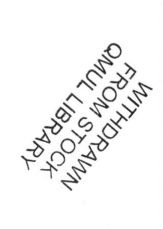

Cutaneous Cryosurgery

Second Edition

Cutaneous Cryosurgery

Principles and Clinical Practice

Second Edition

Rodney Dawber MA, MB ChB, FRCP

Consultant Dermatologist
The Churchill Hospital

Clinical Senior Lecturer in Dermatology
Oxford University
Oxford, UK

Graham Colver DM, MA, BM BCh, FRCP

Consultant Dermatologist
Chesterfield and North Derbyshire Royal Hospital
Chesterfield, UK

Arthur Jackson BSc, MB ChB, MRCGP

Primary Care Physician
Holmes Chapel Health Centre

Clinical Assistant in Dermatology
Leighton Hospital
Crewe, UK

Advisor on Nursing Practice

Fiona Pringle RGN, FETC, FPCert

Surgical Nurse Practitioner
The Churchill Hospital
Oxford, UK

Martin Dunitz

© Martin Dunitz Ltd 1992, 1997

Artwork © Rodney Dawber, Graham Colver and Arthur Jackson 1992

First published in the United Kingdom in 1992,
second edition 1997
by Martin Dunitz Ltd, The Livery House, 7–9 Pratt Street,
London, NW1 0AE

A CIP record for this book is available from the British Library.

ISBN 1 85317 430 0

Composition by Scribe Design, Gillingham, Kent

Originated, printed and bound in Singapore by
Toppan Printing Company (S) Pte Ltd

Contents

Preface

The first edition seems to have found an important place in cryosurgery practice around the world. The specialty has massively expanded in primary care, podiatry and in nursing practice, as nurse-led skin surgery has formally increased. The latter has gathered considerable momentum during the last five years. With this in mind we are pleased to welcome Fiona Pringle to our team. As Secretary of the British Dermatological Nursing Group (affiliated to the British Association of Dermatologists), she has been in the forefront of setting the necessary standards for nurses taking this clinical lead.

In response to comments and constructive criticisms from various colleagues around the world we have in particular modified the practical schedules in the various clinical sections—in order to give relative newcomers to cryosurgery practice 'average' freeze schedules and times for typical lesions in the various diagnostic categories—these are guidelines and in no way 'carved in stone'!

Rodney Dawber
Graham Colver
Arthur Jackson

1 Introduction

Many physical therapies used to treat human disease have a history of gradual evolution. Their introduction may have been on the basis of quasi-scientific reasoning, observation of natural phenomena or serendipity. One example is the surgical treatment of breast cancer which has undergone great changes, in one decade becoming more aggressive and destructive and later being much less so. Another physical treatment that has a long history is phototherapy. The ancient Egyptians were aware of an interaction between the juice of a plant, painted on to the skin, and sunlight. Centuries later we are doing the same in a more controlled manner, the equipment and dosimetry becoming more refined. The science of cryosurgery is no different. Nature has given us wonderful examples of superficial and deep freezing techniques, the lessons learned being that deep destruction is possible, that anaesthesia can result from superficial cooling and that excellent aesthetic results are seen after superficial destruction of tissue in this way.

Cryosurgery literally means cold handiwork. It may be described as the branch of therapeutics that makes use of local freezing for the controlled destruction or removal of living tissue. Before the term 'cryosurgery' came into common usage during the 1960s, various other names were used, including cryocautery, cryocongelation, cryotherapy, cryogenic therapeutics and cryogenic surgery.

The way in which cryosurgery has come of age is discussed in the next chapter. It is widely used, which would seem to indicate that its efficacy is acknowledged and proven. Indeed the most important question which can be asked of any treatment is whether it works. In some ways this is the hardest question to answer and the history of all surgical techniques is studded with conflicting reports. Scalpel surgery for instance had long been the benchmark for treating skin malignancy. But clearly it does not work in all cases because there are some recurrences. Taking wider margins may improve the cure rate but even micrographic surgery, the new gold standard, does not have a 100 per cent success rate. So in answer to the question 'Does scalpel surgery work'? it has to be admitted that usually it does, but there are always some failures. Other studies have shown that even when there is histological evidence of tumour at the excision margin the tumour only recurs in 20 per cent of cases. Comparisons between studies, which deal with cure rates in premalignant and malignant disease, are hampered by minor differences in technique as well as patient and lesion selection. For example, it would not be possible to compare two studies looking at cure rates for

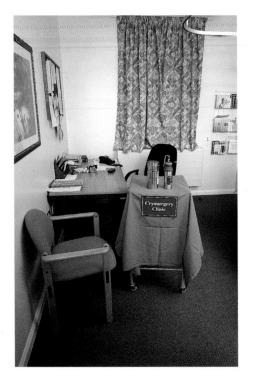

Figure 1.1

A cryosurgery unit.

excision of small basal cell carcinomas if they did not contain the same number of tumours in the high risk areas of the face. One observer may measure the lesions, and the margins for excision, under magnification with operating quality lighting while another may do it by naked eye, and the difference may be significant.

In the field of cryosurgery similar difficulties hamper interpretation of some studies. In the chapter on equipment and techniques attention is drawn to the killing ability of liquid nitrogen and how this is related to temperature, the rapidity of freezing, thaw time and other parameters. Attempts to control these variables include a standardised notation to document the treatment schedule, using the cryospray method with a standard nozzle size, neoprene cones and even thermocouple monitoring. The problem with the latter being that the operator does not know precisely at what depth the thermocouple has been placed. In this book frequent reference is made to the importance of adhering rigorously to a standardised treatment protocol and notation for recording treatment parameters.

Cryosurgery is becoming more sophisticated for two reasons: first that there are now a huge number of studies on clinical efficacy and secondly that the scientific understanding of cryobiology has progressed rapidly. The importance of good studies cannot be overemphasised and fortunately there are now some excellent ones involving large patient numbers and with follow-up to 10 years and more. Many of these studies come from those parts of the world where people with a celtic type skin are living in areas with high ambient ultraviolet levels. The result is a population with an extremely high prevalence of skin malignancy and a large number of individuals have multiple tumours. The local practitioners therefore see more malignancy in a year than some European specialists may see in a lifetime.

Cutaneous cryosurgery is practised not only by most dermatologists in Europe, USA and Australasia but also by a burgeoning number of primary care physicians. Many will use it only for viral warts, solar and seborrhoeic keratoses but others gradually increase their repertoire. It is vital that all operators have an understanding of the scientific aspects of this treatment modality and have supervised clinical experience before going it alone. Some individuals assume that it is a simple business with wide safety margins. It cannot be stressed too much that there is great variability of response in different anatomical sites and between individuals and that liquid nitrogen is a destructive agent.

Safety officers, working in institutions where liquid nitrogen is used industrially, spend much of their time educating employees how to avoid contact with the substance.

The need to educate practitioners before they use cryosurgery has been tackled by the Task Force on Cryosurgery formed by the American Academy of Dermatologists. In their guidelines (1994) they suggest that physicians using cryosurgery should not only have the requisite knowledge but also have attended an appropriate course and have 'experience at the surgical table under the supervision of a physician experienced in this technique'. In the UK the extended role of nurses has naturally led to a number of dermatology and primary care nurses developing their skills and participating or leading cryosurgery sessions. This area is discussed in detail.

This book is a consensus view of busy practitioners. It aims to encourage the thoughtful and appropriate use of liquid nitrogen cryosurgery. While a huge amount of scientific literature has been taken into consideration the aim is to distil that which is relevant to safe, everyday practice. Cryosurgery is certainly widely used. In many instances it is the treatment of choice and for certain benign lesions it is a first rate, quick and cost effective therapy. Its use for cosmetic purposes such as reducing pigmentation or treating areas of sebaceous hyperplasia is increasing and is satisfying to perform. In certain situations it is the treatment of choice for malignant tumours and can be used for palliation in others. It may have particular application in patients receiving anticoagulants, those allergic to local anaesthetics or who have pacemakers or a phobia for needles. Whatever the reason for choosing the liquid nitrogen modality it is crucial that the practitioner has made a firm clinical diagnosis and has discussed with the patient the rationale for the choice. Because clinical diagnosis plays such an important part the book is laid out with an emphasis on

those clinical features to look for in suitable lesions. Chapters 4, 5 and 6 have an atlas of clinical practice which gives visual guidance to the type of lesions being treated and the results which can be expected.

Setting up a cryosurgery clinic

Whether setting up a cryosurgery clinic in hospital practice or a primary care setting, it is important and worthwhile to take the time to make preliminary arrangements and to check back-up services. Such preparations can help to ensure that delays, disappointments or even mistakes are subsequently avoided.

Cryosurgery equipment is not dealt with in this chapter, but is described in detail in Chapter 3.

An eight-point plan can be proposed for setting up a cryosurgery clinic:

- Arrange training for doctor and nurse.
- Arrange a regular supply of liquid nitrogen (see Chapter 3).
- Make arrangements for histology reports.
- Organize provision of biopsy packs, local anaesthetic, suture material, dressings and so on.
- Set aside clinic time for the doctor and nurse.
- Obtain consent and provide information handouts for patients.
- Keep good records of treatment.
- Decide follow-up policy.

Arrange training for doctor and nurse

Cryosurgery—the use of subzero temperature to destroy unwanted tissues—is a relatively new art or subspecialty in hospital practice. Not all hospital dermatology departments undertake cryosurgery. Some that do, limit themselves to treating benign lesions.

Primary care physicians have used cryogens such as carbon dioxide snow for treating warts for many years. The use of liquid nitrogen is now more widespread. In the UK, this is partly because of reimbursements made for minor surgery procedures listed in the 1990 General Practitioner Contract. It is essential, in these circumstances, that the biological basis for cryosurgery is properly understood.

Liquid nitrogen has the lowest boiling point (–196°C) of all the available refrigerants and is the cryogen of choice. A sound knowledge of cryobiology is essential, however, before undertaking treatment of skin lesions, particularly where malignancy is concerned.

Simple and benign skin lesions can be treated by a single freeze followed by a natural thaw—a single freeze–thaw cycle.

Malignant skin lesions require a 25–30 second freeze, a minimum 5 minute thaw, followed in most cases by another 25–30 second freeze—a double freeze–thaw cycle.

Practitioners in hospital or in primary health care starting out in cryosurgery can first gain valuable experience by attending dermatological surgery workshops. Here aspects of skin surgery and cryosurgery techniques can be learned using pigs' feet as models. Where dermatology departments have cryosurgery clinics, sitting in on such clinics is of great value to practitioners building up their experience in the cryosurgery field. Clearly, such practitioners should personally gain experience in treating benign lesions before progressing to treatment of malignant lesions.

In the setting up and running of a cryosurgery clinic, the nurse plays a crucial role. Even when the doctor carrying out the cryosurgery has explained the procedure, its effects and outcome to the patient, the nurse has a role in further communication and reassurance to the patient. The nurse's skills are invaluable during the procedure and vital in the aftercare of the wound, whether in a hospital clinic or in primary health care. It is therefore important to encourage nurses to attend cryosurgery workshops or meetings with their medical colleagues. This ensures that their skills can be used to the full and an efficient cryosurgery service can be offered.

Nurses carrying out nurse-led cryosurgery clinics for the treatment of warts and other benign skin lesions must be adequately trained and fully competent. No treatment should be undertaken if the diagnosis of the lesion is in doubt. Back-up medical care must always be available.

Arrange a regular supply of liquid nitrogen

Liquid nitrogen is now readily available. Most hospitals have storage capacity and suitable containers or storage flasks for use in a cryosurgery clinic. Fewer primary health care centres, however, have storage facilities for liquid nitrogen.

It is essential to organize a reliable source of liquid nitrogen if one is to run a regular cryosurgery clinic in primary medicine. This can be done in one of several ways. If a primary care physician can provide a suitable portable storage flask and protective container, the local hospital is usually happy to provide the liquid nitrogen required at a reasonable cost. Several firms in the UK involved in the supply of cryosurgery equipment offer a built-in supply service at an annual cost for the liquid nitrogen and for the rental of storage equipment. For the practitioner who is very involved in cryosurgery in primary health care, a large 35 litre or 50 litre storage flask is available which can be topped

GUIDANCE NOTES
Transport by vehicle of liquid nitrogen in containers of less than 450 litres capacity

SCOPE

These guidance notes are for the user of portable cryogenic vessels of less than 450 litres capacity. These guidance notes do not substitute any part of the statutory regulations where they apply to certain vessels.

VESSELS

Any vessel used should be vacuum insulated and in good condition. The vessel must have provision for venting gas that boils off from the liquid. Vessels should be labelled, indicating the contents and the potential hazards.

LOADING

The liquid nitrogen vessel should, where possible, be carried in an open vehicle or trailer. If this is not possible and the container is to be transported in the passenger compartment (including the book area) then consideration must be given to the risk of asphyxiation. Whatever the position of loading the vessel must ALWAYS be secured in an upright position and NOT HELD BY HAND. Open dewars containing more than 0.3 litres should not be carried in the passenger compartment.

HAZARDS

Carriage of liquid nitrogen within a vehicle may lead to potential hazards from escape of gas or spillage of very cold liquid nitrogen. The significant hazards are:

a) Spillage of cryogenic liquids can cause cold burns, frost bite or hypothermia. Spillage also releases gas into the atmosphere. For example, one volume of liquid will release 683 times that volume of gas.

b) Release of gas can cause a dramatic change in the surrounding atmosphere. Release of nitrogen can cause oxygen deficiency and lead to asphyxis of personnel in the area. An atmosphere containing less than 18% oxygen is potentially hazardous and entry into atmospheres containing less than 20% oxygen should be avoided.

All cryogenic liquid storage vessels will produce gas as a result of normal heat in leak through the vacuum insulation. Generally 1% to 2% of the liquid content is converted to gas in 24 hours. When open dewars, refrigerators or other non-pressurised vessels are used this gas will enter the atmosphere creating a potential hazard in a confined space. In pressure vessels this gas builds up until the relief valve pressure is reached, at which point the valve opens and allows gas to vent to atmosphere, the valve will reset when the pressure falls below the relief valve set pressure. In the unlikely event that the relief valve is unable to cope with a rapid build up of pressure the burst disc will rupture once the pressure reaches the design failure pressure. When the disc bursts the decrease in pressure will result in rapid boil off of liquid and venting of the pressurised gas. Similarly in the event of vessel failure due to impact or other cause all gas will be released rapidly to atmosphere.

PRECAUTIONS

Always ensure that:

1. Ventilation is adequate to maintain the atmosphere at 20.8% oxygen concentration - use a fan and ventilation from the outside air and open windows. An oxygen monitor should be used to detect nitrogen enrichment. The positioning of the monitor should be away from any ventilation source.
2. Pressure vessels are fully depressurised prior to transport and all valves are fully closed.
3. Passengers and drivers are not liable to be splashed with liquid from any open dewar in the event of a collision and the vessel is fully secured away from any potential impact.

To calculate the worst scenario, refer to BOC Guidance Notes for users of liquid cylinders of low pressure cryogenic liquid suply vessels - G4521 2.90.

EMERGENCY ACTIONS

In the event that liquid spills from an open dewar while being transported, the window closet to the driver and any passengers should be fully opened to ventilate the vehicle and provide air to the occupants. The vehicle should be parked in an area that will not cause a hazard and the spilt liquid allowed to boil off and ventilate from the vehicle (open all doors and windows to assist this). All occupants should leave the vehicle.

Should a pressure vessel reach the relief valve set pressure and gas escape (see 'precautions 2') the vehicle should be immediately ventilated and vehicle parked in a safe area that will not cause a hazard. All occupants should leave the vehicle. When safe to do so the vessel should be removed from the vehicle and fully depressurised, checking for the cause of the rise in pressure (this may have been caused by the pressure raising valve being activated). Providing the pressure can be reduced the vessel may be reloaded, secured and the journey continued with caution.

Note: Under the Health and Safety at Work Act 1974 a safe system of work should be adopted where practical when a potential hazard has been identified.

BOC Cryospeed can provide a point of use delivery service of small quantities of liquid nitrogen to avoid personal risk.

ADDITIONAL BOC REFERENCES

Care with Cryogenics G2246.
Prevention of Oxygen Enrichment or Deficiency Accident G4256.
Treatment of Cryogenic Burns & Frostbite G4968.
Nitrogen Data & Safety Sheet G4095.
BOC Cryospeed Liquid Nitrogen G4292.

ASPHYXIATION WARNING: LIQUID NITROGEN IS A RISK TO LIFE WHEN TRANSPORTED INSIDE A PASSENGER VEHICLE

up at appropriate intervals on a cost per litre basis by a local supplier.

Make arrangements for histology reports

The basis of good, safe cryosurgery is pretreatment histopathology where malignancy is suspected or the histology is in doubt. Before one undertakes cryosurgery in primary care medicine, therefore, it is necessary to confirm that good histopathology services are available. Any specimen submitted should be sent in a container of buffered formalin, normally provided by the hospital pathology department. The container must be properly labelled and the pathology request card should include the following information:

- Name, date of birth and address of patient;
- Name and address of doctor;
- Short history of lesion;
- Site and type of biopsy (e.g. incision edge biopsy, curettage biopsy or excision biopsy);
- Histology required.

Organize provision of biopsy packs, local anaesthetic, suture material, dressings and so on

Biopsy packs

The contents of a biopsy pack are often a matter of personal choice. Table 1.1 lists the contents of a suitable biopsy pack (see also Figure 1.2).

In addition the following may be necessary: a no. 15 scalpel blade for full thickness, incisional biopsy, or a 2 or 3 mm biopsy punch if a punch biopsy is considered suitable.

Chlorhexidine gluconate 0.05 per cent is a suitable solution (25 ml sachet) for preparation and cleansing of a biopsy site.

Local anaesthetic

The 'safe dose' of local anaesthetic for skin infiltration is: 20 ml of lignocaine (1 per cent) or 10 ml of lignocaine (2 per cent).

The addition of adrenaline reduces toxicity by half thus doubling the safe dose, i.e. 40 ml of lignocaine (1 per cent with adrenaline 1 in 200 000); 20 ml of lignocaine (2 per cent with adrenaline 1 in 200 000).

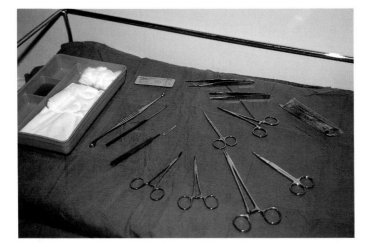

Figure 1.2

Biopsy pack, set out.

Table 1.1   Contents of a biopsy pack.

1 Scalpel handle (Bard–Parker) No. 3
1 Spencer Wells forceps
2 Curved mosquito forceps
1 Pair of straight pointed scissors
1 Pair of strabismus scissors
1 Kilner or Mayo needle holder
1 Non-toothed dissecting forceps
1 McIndoe's fine dissecting forceps
1 Gillies skin hook
1 Volkmann's spoon (medium)
5 Cotton-wool balls
10 Gauze swabs (7.5 cm × 7.5 cm)
5 Regal swabs (10 cm × 10 cm)
2 Theatre towels

Also available is a very useful pre-filled dental cartridge containing 2.2 ml lignocaine 2 per cent with adrenaline 1 in 80 000. A similar cartridge containing 2.2 ml of prilocaine (4 per cent) equivalent to lignocaine (2 per cent without adrenaline) can be used for digital anaesthesia. Both local anaesthetic cartridges fit into a dental syringe to which can be fitted a fine, flexible dental needle which makes cutaneous anaesthesia easier, with fewer puncture sites than with the conventional, rigid needle.

Lignocaine 2.5 per cent, prilocaine 2.5 per cent (EMLA) cream may be used for surface anaesthesia, particularly when treating warts or molluscum contagiosum in younger children. This should be applied two hours before treatment.

Suture material

Polyglycolate or polygalactin absorbable sutures for subcutaneous use.

Ethilon 4/0 (W319), Ethilon 3/0 (W320) or Ethilon 6/0 (W507). Alternatively there is Prolene 4/0 (W539)—these are all non-absorbable sutures for cutaneous use.

Mersilk should be used for scalp or mucous membranes only. Mersilk is too abrasive for routine skin suturing and inevitably causes some local reaction which makes for less than good cosmetic results.

Other pieces of equipment essential to the cryosurgeon are: a magnifying lens to define the full extent of the lesion; a marker pen to outline the area to be treated; and a simple ruler to record the size of the lesion.

Set aside clinic time for the doctor and nurse

If an efficient, well-equipped cutaneous surgery/cryosurgery clinic is to be run in the best interest of both doctor and patient, it is essential to set aside time which is both adequate and suitable: 'suitable' in that it must be a time at which a trained nurse can assist and that all the equipment necessary is available; 'adequate' in at which it will be sufficient for treating the number of patients intended. As a guide, in a 2–3 hour session 5–8 patients might be treated, depending on their lesions. The frequency of the clinics will obviously depend on the demand—possibly weekly in hospital and monthly in primary health care.

Obtain consent and provide information handouts for patients

However good the doctor's rapport with a patient, consent cannot be implied when undertaking cryosurgery. The consent form (Figure 1.3) need not be elaborate, but for legal purposes must be signed by the patient (or guardian if the patient is a child) and the doctor carrying out the procedures.

Before seeking consent, it is very important to explain to the patient the details of cryosurgical treatment in terms of:

- The aims of the treatment;
- The possible effects from the treatment in terms of initial swelling and other side-effects;
- The subsequent changes and care of the treated area;
- The probable cosmetic outcome of treatment;
- The follow-up arrangements, especially when dealing with malignant lesions.

In addition to discussing the procedure with the patient, a simple handout explaining the effects of treatment is very helpful and reassuring to the patient (see Tables 4.1 and 6.3).

Keep good records of treatment

For legal, audit and research purposes accurate records should be kept regarding each cryosurgery procedure carried out. Details should include:

- Name, date of birth and address of the patient;
- Date of treatment;
- Type of lesion, size and site;
- Local anaesthetic used;
- Any sutures used when carrying out a biopsy;
- Exact procedure carried out (e.g. double 25 second freeze–thaw cycle using liquid nitrogen cryospray), nozzle size and distance from skin;
- Complications, if any;

- Topical application and dressing used;
- Nurse assistant present;
- Doctor carrying out the procedure.

Space for definitive histopathology should also be available.

All these details are best kept in a proper cryosurgery/surgical procedures book. Separate records of each patient should also be kept for reference and subsequent follow-up.

Decide follow-up policy

All patients undergoing cryosurgery treatment must have follow-up appropriate to the lesion that has been treated.

Initial wound care following cryosurgery can well be looked after and supervised by the clinic nurse. However, the doctor embarking on cryosurgery would benefit from being involved at this stage in order to observe the progress of treatment. Any problems or side-effects should be recorded.

It is instructive and helpful to doctor and patient alike to check the cryosurgery wound at 6–8 weeks. This provides a useful opportunity to assess the clinical and cosmetic outcome of treatment and to discuss any problems with the patient.

Until one becomes familiar with the outcome of cryosurgery in the treatment of malignant lesions, in addition to the checks outlined above it is a good policy to review patients at 6, 12, 18 months and 2 years. These reviews are to assess the outcome and to exclude any recurrences. Patients should also be encouraged to report to their primary care physician at any time should they be concerned about changes at the treatment site or any new skin lesions.

A nurse-led cryosurgery service

Several questions need to be addressed before commencing a nurse-led cryosurgery clinic:

- Why do you want a nurse to perform cryosurgery?
- Who is going to train the nurse?
- What time-scale for training is being allowed?
- Will the nurse-led clinic receive secretarial support?
- Does the nurse have indemnity cover either from a union or hospital trust?
- What nursing roles will the nurse have to give up in order to run a cryosurgery service?
- Will it benefit the patients if a nurse runs a cryosurgery clinic?

The profession of nursing is undergoing immense change. The introduction of extended roles and nurse practitioners is coinciding with a reduction in junior doctors hours and an emphasis on their training. The boundaries between the two disciplines are being eroded in many areas including dermatology.

Cryosurgery is relatively easy, quick and cheap to perform whether in a primary or secondary health care setting. It is a field in which nurses can become expert practitioners. Already many nurses successfully run cryosurgery clinics, treating patients with a variety of conditions. However if nursing is to remain dynamic, then thought must be given to the training needs of nurses new to the specialty.

Accountability

The Patients Charter (1991) in the UK encourages patients to exercise their rights to high quality care; it is therefore vital to ensure the appropriate training and competence of individuals carrying out dermatological procedures. Nurses are governed by the UKCC (United Kingdom Central Council for Nursing, Midwifery and Health Visiting) and bound by their Code of Professional Conduct. Registered nurses are personally accountable for their practice which must therefore be sensitive, relevant and respond to the needs of individual patients. The range of responsibilities which fall to individual nurses should relate to their personal experience, education and skill.

In 1992 the UKCC published the Scope of Professional Practice document. It states that, in any role the nurse must be satisfied that all aspects of practice are directed to meeting the needs and serving the interests of patients. Also, the registered nurse must:

- endeavour to achieve and develop knowledge, skill and competence to respond to those needs and interests;
- honestly acknowledge any limits of personal knowledge and skill and take steps to remedy any relevant deficits in order to meet the needs of patients;
- ensure that any enlargement or adjustment of the scope of practice must be achieved without compromising or fragmenting existing aspects of patient care;
- recognise and honour the direct or indirect personal accountability for all aspects of professional practice;
- in serving the interests of patients and the wider interests of society, avoid any inappropriate delegation to others which compromises those interests.

This last statement means that managers cannot expect nurses to take on new roles without adequate training and nurses must, in the interest of their patients, say if they are not happy with any area of their workload.

In effect, the nurse as an accountable practitioner has the right to agree to do anything and refuse to do everything!

Table 1.2   Clinical assessment criteria.

	Level of achievement	*Grade*
Novice	Cannot perform this activity satisfactorily to participate in the clinical environment	0
	Can perform this activity but not without constant supervision and some assistance	1
	Can perform this activity satisfactorily but requires some supervision and assistance	2
Competent Practitioner	Can perform this activity satisfactorily without assistance and/or supervision	3
	Can perform this activity satisfactorily without supervision or assistance with more than acceptable speed and quality of work	4
	Can perform this activity satisfactorily with more than acceptable speed and quality and with initiative and adaptability to special problem situations	5
Clinical Expert	Can perform this activity with more than acceptable speed and quality, with initiative and adaptability and can lead others in performing this task	6

The training

Training for undertaking cryosurgery should be given by an appropriately qualified practitioner. This may be a consultant dermatologist in the case of hospital based nurses or a primary care physician with a specialist interest in dermatology in the case of community based staff.

Theoretical knowledge should be consolidated with a period of observation in a cryosurgery clinic. Once the learner and trainer are confident of the nurse's ability, the nurse should then undertake a period of supervised practice. The length of time of this practice will vary, depending on the confidence and skill of the nurse and the level of competence achieved.

Guidelines for use of the competency framework

- Having identified an appropriate mentor/supervisor for the period of supervised practice, an initial assessment, using the clinical assessment criteria (Tables 1.2 and 1.3) is made. The grades are entered in the grids provided underneath the specific competencies for the given skill and this is then dated and signed.
- When it is deemed mutually appropriate between mentor and learner, following a period of supervision, a secondary assessment is performed. The new grades are entered into the grid and then an arrow inserted to denote an increase or decrease in grade for the secondary assessment.

Table 1.3 Competencies for performing cryosurgery.

Demonstrates knowledge of the structure and function of the skin

☐☐☐☐☐☐

Effectively prepares the patient physically and psychologically for the procedure

☐☐☐☐☐☐

Safely and effectively performs the cryosurgery using a Cry-ac flask

☐☐☐☐☐☐

Can select appropriate dressings for the site and conveys any after care required to the patient effectively

☐☐☐☐☐☐

Understands the indications for performing cryosurgery

☐☐☐☐☐☐

Can state the possible complications of local anaesthetic administration and their significance

☐☐☐☐☐☐

Demonstrates knowledge of freeze-thaw cycles and their function

☐☐☐☐☐☐

Demonstrates knowledge of use of steroids and their side-effects and their use post cryosurgery

☐☐☐☐☐☐

Selects and prepares appropriate equipment for cryosurgery

☐☐☐☐☐☐

Selects a suitable size nozzle for the cryo-gun and discuss reasons for that choice

☐☐☐☐☐☐

Can state possible complications of cryosurgery

☐☐☐☐☐☐

Demonstrates accurate recording of events in patient's record and the operation register

☐☐☐☐☐☐

Date of initial assessment: . . . .

Signature of mentor/supervisor: . . . .

Date of secondary assessment: . . . .

Signature of mentor/supervisor: . . . .

Date of tertiary assessment: . . . .

Signature of mentor/supervisor: . . . .

Date of subsequent assessment: . . . .

Signature of mentor/supervisor: . . . .

Example:
Is able to correctly and safely fill and prepare the cryospray equipment for use.
  – initial assessment = 1
  – secondary assessment = 2

• The tertiary assessment is performed as above.
• When learners are identified as having reached grade 3 for all the competencies, they are deemed safe to practise without supervision. The number of assessments required to reach grade 3 will be individual. Prior to independent practise the learner must inform the clinical nurse manager of their intent to practise.
• The learner must at all times uphold the UKCC Code of Professional Conduct.

CONSENT FORM   APPENDIX A (3)

For treatment by a health professional other than doctors or dentists

Health Authority ....   Patient's Surname ....

Hospital ....   Other Names ....

Unit Number ....   Date of Birth ....

Sex: *(please tick)*   Male ☐   Female ☐

HEALTH PROFESSIONAL *(This part to be completed by health professional. See notes on the reverse)*

TYPE OF TREATMENT PROPOSED

Complete this part of the form
I confirm that I have explained the treatment proposed and such appropriate options as are available to the patient in terms which in my judgement are suited to the understanding of the patient and/or to one of the parents or guardians of the patient.

Signature ....Date ..../................/ ....

Name of health professional ....

Job title of health professional ....

PATIENT/PARENT/GUARDIAN

1. Please read this form and the notes overleaf very carefully.

2. If there is anything that you don't understand about the explanation, or if you want more information, you should ask the health professional who has explained the treatment proposed.

3. Please check that all the information on the form is correct. If it is, and you understand the treatment proposed, then sign the form.

   I am the patient/parent/guardian *(delete as necessary)*

   I agree   ■ to what is proposed which has been explained to me by the health professional named on this form.

Signature ....

Name ....

Address ....

(if not the patient) ....

Figure 1.3

Patient information sheet/patient operation sheet with space for signature for consent to the procedure.

Patient selection

All patients should see a doctor initially to confirm diagnosis prior to treatment. Legally nurses cannot diagnose a patient's condition. Once the diagnosis has been confirmed either by diagnostic biopsy or on examination by a dermatologist or a primary care physician with experience in dermatology, the patient can be referred on to be treated by the nurse.

Patient consent

There are several issues surrounding patient consent, not the least of which is whether it is really necessary. The procedure should be fully explained prior to obtaining the patient's written consent. The nurse carrying out the cryosurgery should be the one to obtain the patient's consent.

Patient care

Patient education is an important part of the nurse's role. The nurse will be able to advise the patient on wound care and any further treatment that may be required, ideally giving written guidelines on post cryosurgery care. The patient should know how to contact the department again, if necessary.

Prescribing

Some practitioners use local anaesthetic before cryosurgery. In those cases Lignocaine 1% will be administered. Following cryosurgery Dermovate ointment is sometimes used to reduce the post-inflammatory reaction. Nurse prescribing is not yet standard practice in either the hospital or primary care setting: local policies will need to be drawn up. It is advisable to work closely with your local pharmacist. The training programme will need to include the use and side-effects of both local anaesthesia and topical steroids.

Monitoring and auditing

To ensure that the service is effective in meeting the needs of patients, it will need to be monitored. This can be done in several ways. The number of visits required to treat viral warts effectively can be audited. The recurrence rate for viral warts can be monitored. There must be a commitment on the part of both the nurse and the nurse manager to continuing education, by attendance at relevant study days and courses. The nurse's performance and training needs should be monitored and appraised six monthly.

Resource implications

To be most effective, the nurse should perform cryosurgery in a designated clinic. Ideally, there should always be a doctor available for advice whilst the clinic is in progress. The development of nurse-led cryosurgery clinics can help relieve the pressure on waiting lists for outpatient appointments. There is often improved continuity of care for patients especially if they had previously normally attended a large teaching hospital department.

Bibliography

Burge S, Colver G, Lester R (1996), *Simple skin surgery, second edition* (Oxford, Blackwell).

Jackson AD (1995), Prevention, early detection and team management of skin cancer in primary care: contribution to *The health of the nation* objectives, *B J Gen Pract*, **45**: 97–101.

Guidelines of care for cryosurgery (1994), *J Am Acad Dermatol* **31**(**4**): 648–653.

2 Historical and scientific basis of cryosurgery

The nature of cold

Cooling can best be described as the withdrawal of heat. Many factors influence the rate of removal of heat but one of the most important is the proximity to the source of heat removal (i.e. cold object). Slow cooling is not as harmful to tissue as rapid cooling. Indeed, ultraslow reduction in temperature has been used medically for heart and brain operations. Different cells, tissues and organisms have their own susceptibility to cold. At one extreme there are viruses that can survive for years in liquid nitrogen at −196°C. Human cells, however, do not survive this degree of cold. Different cell lines die at particular temperatures and several parameters will affect that temperature, e.g. concomitant vascular effects; but there is a minimum below which cells will die and in the skin this is generally around −30 to −40°C.

The fact that skin lesions are visible has always meant that inquisitive Man has been able to experiment in an empirical, pragmatic way, using a variety of chemical or physical treatments—fashion and whim have at times been the guiding principle. He was also clearly able to observe the effects of different natural physical phenomena on skin, such as

heat, light and cold. In this way over several thousand years, a mass of anecdotal information has been handed down. Long before the measurement and scientific 'objectivity' of the last 150 years, the effects of cold on skin were well described. For example, the eminent medical practitioner John Hunter of London in 1777 stated, from observations long before the age of in vitro studies, animal models and detailed microscopy of post-treatment biopsies, that 'The local tissue response to freezing includes local tissue necrosis, vascular stasis and excellent healing' (quoted in Dawber, 1988)—virtually the whole basis and conclusions of cryobiology and cryosurgery succinctly and clearly expounded over 200 years ago!

In a review of the historical evolution of cryosurgery, three fields can be delineated—the use of cold from natural sources, the production of refrigerants colder than ice by 'modern' physical science during the last 150 years, and biological and clinical research into the effects of extreme cold on normal and diseased skin (Figures 2.1–2.3). Clinical progress could not have evolved into such an efficacious branch of surgery without the interplay of knowledge from these three areas.

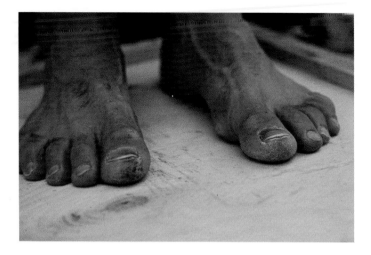

Figure 2.1

Cyanosis and incipient gangrene of both great toes after high-altitude mountain climbing without oxygen.

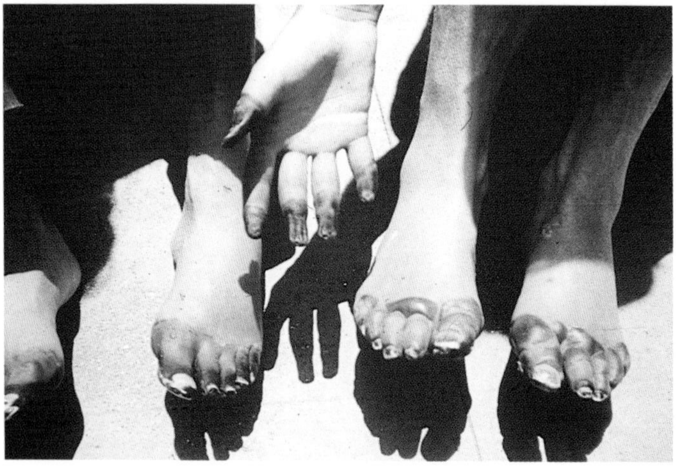

Figure 2.2

Gangrene of toes and fingers of two climbers following prolonged high-altitude exposure.

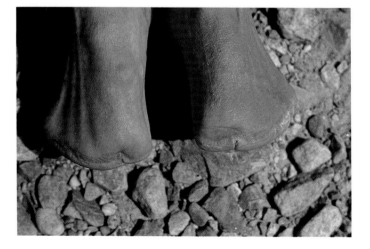

Figure 2.3

Same toes as Figure 2.2 – 2 years later.

The use of cold in medicine dates back over 4000 years to the ancient Egyptians. They noted that the application of cold minimized the pain of trauma and decreased inflammation. Hippocrates recommended hypothermia to reduce swelling, haemorrhage and pain and observed that it had local anaesthetic properties (see Dawber, 1988). These findings were confirmed by the physician-surgeon, Dominique Jean Larrey, the military surgeon of Napoleon's army during the historic and tragic retreat from Moscow. He found that the injured limbs of wounded soldiers could be amputated with minimum pain and haemorrhage if the limb was covered with ice or snow before the operation. He stated that 'Cold acts by reducing the sensibility of those organs that are under immediate attack. Cold has a sedatory affect which acts, above all, on the brain and nervous system' (quoted in Dawber, 1988).

James Arnott of London pioneered refrigeration local analgesia for the treatment of a variety of surface conditions, including the palliation of cancerous tumours in terminally ill patients (Arnott, 1851). He achieved temperatures of –24°C by employing a solution of ice and saline. He attained considerable fame and demonstrated his equipment at the Great Exhibition of London in 1851. He is often described as the father of 'modern' cryosurgery.

Zacarian (1985) dates the birth of modern cryogenics to the year 1877. Two papers were delivered before the French Academy of Sciences, one by a French scientist, Cailletet, and the second by a Swiss engineer, Pictet. Cailletet described the liquefaction of small quantities of oxygen and carbon monoxide by expansion of the gases from extremely high pressures. Pictet demonstrated the liquefaction of oxygen by means of a mechanical refrigeration cascade, employing sulphur dioxide and carbon dioxide boiled under reduced pressures. Six years later in Poland, Wroblewski and Olszewski converted oxygen and nitrogen into the liquid state. The commercial production of liquid air and the extraction from it of liquid nitrogen was carried out by Linde shortly before 1900. On recognizing the Joule–Thompson expansion principle (in which cooling occurs when a gas is expanded from a high pressure), Dewar liquefied hydrogen in 1898 and also developed the vacuum flask for the storage and transport of cryogenic fluids. This was a very significant advance in that it enabled the clinician to have such liquids readily available for use in clinical practice.

The first significant use of extremely cold refrigerants (liquefied air) for medical disorders is attributed to White in 1899. He trained in dermatology and was a clinician with an investigative curiosity. He initially dipped cotton-tipped applicators into liquefied air and reported the successful treatment of warts, naevi and various precancerous skin conditions. He also treated many malignant tumours of the skin with good results, stating 'I can truly say today that I believe that epithelioma treated early in its existence by liquid air, will always be cured, and that many inoperable cases can also be cured by its application' (White, 1901). Bowen and Towle used liquid air for the treatment of pigmented hairy naevi, various vascular skin lesions, such as port-wine and cavernous haemangiomas and lymphangioma (see Dawber, 1988). By this time it was already being noted that cryosurgery healing showed less scarring potential and often gave better cosmetic results than other surgical methods of treatment. In 1907, Whitehouse, a New York dermatologist, devised a method to spray the refrigerant. The spray was obtained by inserting a rubber cork pierced by two glass tubes in an ordinary laboratory wash-bottle, the mouth of the entering tube being closed by the finger. He successfully treated many patients with skin carcinomas using this equipment. Whitehouse did, however, find this equipment difficult to use in practice, expressing a preference for the cotton-swab dip method.

Contemporary with the use of liquid air, many authorities were diligently experimenting with the clinical uses of carbon dioxide snow. The most eminent proponent of this was William Pusey of Chicago, who emphasized the ready availability of carbon dioxide, because of its widespread use wherever soda-fountain supplies were sold. Whitehouse had shown that liquid air could be used in swab form or spray to treat a vast array of benign skin lesions; Pusey (1907) promoted carbon dioxide (carbonic acid) snow to be used in a similar way. The use of the latter was much more popular in Europe—Cranston Low of Edinburgh (1911) and Hall-Edwards of Birmingham, England (1913) produced small monographs extolling its virtues. That Hall-Edwards was writing in this field was remarkable in that he was primarily a very eminent and experienced radiotherapist at a time when irradiation was finding more and more uses in dermatology.

Between 1920 and 1945, few advances occurred in the field, for many reasons. In relation to cryosurgery specifically, no significant technological or refrigerant advances were made and carbon dioxide snow continued to be the main agent used, usually compacted into sticks or pencils of varying diameter for direct application to the lesion. A modification of this theme was the use in the late 1930s of a mixture of carbon dioxide snow and acetone (carbon dioxide 'slush'). This was used particularly for acne and superficial post-acne scarring. It caused mild erythema and exfoliation. Some dermatologists still use carbon dioxide slush in cosmetic or aesthetic medical practice.

The other main reasons for the lack of progress in the spread of cryosurgical practice were:

- The increasing successes obtained by the use of irradiation—most dermatologists in advanced cultures possessed their own machines and the long-term sequelae were not yet well enough recognized to limit this modality, even for many benign dermatoses;
- The increasing sophistication of excisional surgery and the relative safety of general anaesthesia.

After 1945, liquid nitrogen and oxygen became freely available. Oxygen was little used, mainly for safety reasons, whilst liquid nitrogen became increasingly popular. In its early years, it was only used with the cotton-wool swab method. However, during the 1960s many pressurized liquid nitrogen spray machines were devised which were based on the idea of Whitehouse's spray apparatus. They were of two main types: large, fixed, tabletop machines and handheld portable ones. Much of the credit for developing and popularizing such equipment should go to Zacarian. Many of the spray machines which are used worldwide still look similar to the original units, although they are typically more compact. As liquid nitrogen spray equipment was gaining popularity, a major technical development was produced by Irving Cooper of New York (Cooper, 1963). He described a unit in which liquid nitrogen was circulated through a hollow metal probe that was vacuum-insulated except for its tip. With this equipment it was possible, by interrupting the flow of liquid nitrogen, to control the temperature of the tip within the range of room temperature down to $-196°C$, the boiling point of liquid nitrogen (Table 2.1). Cooper's initial equipment has had a major impact in the treatment of many internal diseases, particularly in neurosurgery, and in the treatment of a variety of tumours such as carcinomas of the prostate and uterine cervix, and hepatic metastasis. Much of the early equipment developed for internal use was far too bulky, complicated and expensive for routine use in dermatology practice. However, almost every liquid nitrogen spray unit developed during the last 20 years has a range of probes, usually copper, through which liquid nitrogen can be circulated and

Table 2.1   Surface tissue temperature reductions attainable with various refrigerants.

Refrigerant	Temperature (°C)
Ice	0°
Salt-Ice	–20°
CO_2 Snow	–79°
CO_2 Slush	–20°
Nitrous oxide	–75°
Liquid nitrogen	–20° (swab)
	–196° (spray or probe)

expelled through a lateral side-arm tube as the gas. Such cooled copper probes have never attained the same popularity as the simple spray, but they are still of considerable use, most commonly for certain benign, nodular, well-circumscribed skin lesions (see Chapters 4, 5 and 6 on treatment methods).

The only other significant technological advance, some 35 years ago, was the innovation by Amoils which used the cooling generated by the Joule–Thompson effect. Amoils' initial equipment was used in ophthalmology (e.g. for lens extractions); but for a variety of reasons, machines using the principle have never attained the same popularity as liquid nitrogen spray and probe units. The main reasons are that the gas cylinders need to be available, careful contact with the lesion ('iceball' formation) is necessary, the rate of fall of temperature is slow and the Joule–Thompson effect is unable to produce 'cancer-killing' low temperatures. However, nitrous oxide probe (Joule–Thompson effect) equipment is still widely used in gynaecology, oral surgery and ophthalmological practice.

All the above advances in cryosurgery, mainly between 1850 and 1960, have related to improvements in refrigeration technology and the harnessing of low temperatures for routine clinical practice. The last 30 years have seen major advances in understanding the biological basis of cryosurgery. The effects of freeze-thaw schedules on normal and pathological skin as heat is withdrawn and returns have been extensively studied.

Shape of the cryolesion

When early workers wanted to look at the shape of the iceball induced by their refrigerants they used gelatin, potatoes and other inanimate models. It soon became apparent that these findings could not be extrapolated to living tissues, principally because a blood supply has a profound effect upon the spread of cold.

Studies to elucidate the relationship between surface temperature, lateral spread and depth of freeze have relied on devices to monitor temperature. These also play a part in clinical practice and they are discussed later in this chapter.

When a tissue is cooled the rate of heat exchange depends on water content, blood supply, thermal conductivity of the tissue, rate of freeze and the temperature of the refrigerant, amongst other variables. There are no simple formulae and further study is still required to produce ideal treatment protocols for the reproducible, consistent destruction of benign and malignant tumours. Much of the information accrued to date, which has led to the present state of the art, comes from experimental work on, for example, pigskin, with temperature monitoring and histological assessment.

The important data that have led to the modern approach to cryosurgical practice can be summarized as follows:

- An open spray (with or without neoprene cones) gives a more rapid drop in temperature and will freeze to a greater depth than a closed probe. However, the shape of the cryolesion is similar for the two methods.

- Down to depths of about 6 mm the contour of the cryolesion is rounded but below this it becomes more triangular in shape (Figure 2.4).
- The lateral spread of ice from the edge of the probe or cone is approximately equal to the depth of freeze (Figure 2.5).
- The isotherms lie closer together when the rate of freezing is rapid. This means that lethal temperatures are found near to the base of the iceball after rapid freezing.
- An open spray was used on live pigskin with thermocouple monitoring. With a surface icefield 2 cm in diameter, maintained for 30 seconds, temperatures below –40°C were recorded at the periphery. Depth measurements gave readings below –50°C at least 5 mm below the surface (Figure 2.6).
- Of the common basal cell carcinomas 90 per cent are 3 mm or less in depth; on the whole the cryosurgical techniques described in this book are recommended for such tumours. The experimental data support the concept that lethal temperatures can be readily achieved at this depth. Because of the relationship between depth and lateral freeze we advocate that the minimum diameter of the icefield should be about 16 mm. This diameter does of course include a margin of healthy skin on either side of the tumour (normally between 3 and 5 mm, depending on the size and type of tumour). As discussed in Chapter 6, we recommend maintaining the established icefield for 30 seconds.

Similar general conclusions have been reached by other authorities in the field; stressing the importance of lateral spread of freeze and rapid cooling, they felt that when treating lesions 0.5–2.5 cm in diameter, a lateral spread of freeze beyond the tumour margin of 5 mm, produced within 60–90 seconds *from the commencement of spraying*, will give a –50°C isotherm depth of about 3 mm.

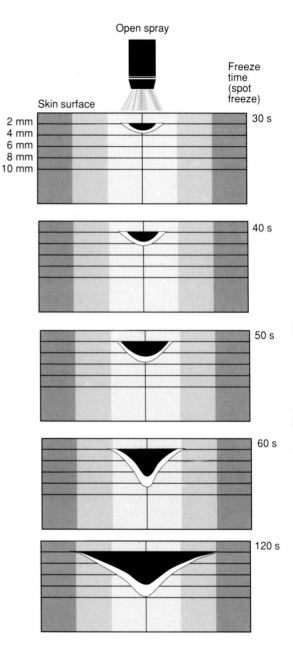

Figure 2.4

Shape of icefield (after Breitbart and Dachów-Siwiéc, 1990).

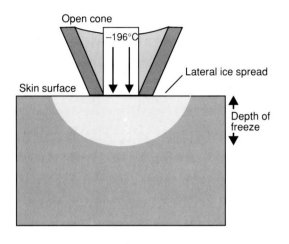

Figure 2.5

Shape of icefield (ball). Note that lateral ice spread is approximately equal to depth of freeze.

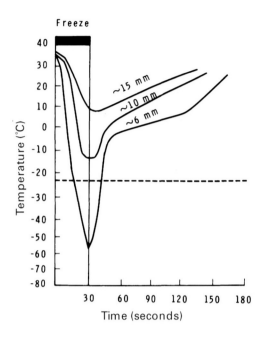

Figure 2.6

Temperatures attained at several depths below a spot freeze of 30 s after icefield formation.

Differential sensitivity of cells

The mechanisms of cell death are described in the next section but different cell lines have their own susceptibility to cold injury. Thus melanocytes are readily damaged by low temperatures whereas fibroblasts are hardy (Figures 2.7–2.11). This has important clinical implications. People with dark or black skin may develop hypopigmentation at the site of freezing. On the other hand, deep freezes, required to treat tumours, are unlikely to destroy the subjacent connective tissue. Table 2.2 shows the relative sensitivities of some cells, organisms and tissues to low temperatures.

Table 2.2   Relative sensitivities to low temperatures.

Cell/tissue/organism	Sensitivity
Melanocytes	Sensitive to cold injury (easily killed)
Basal cells Keratinocytes Bacteria Connective tissue Neural connective tissue sheath Blood vessel endothelium Viruses	↓
	Insensitive to cold injury

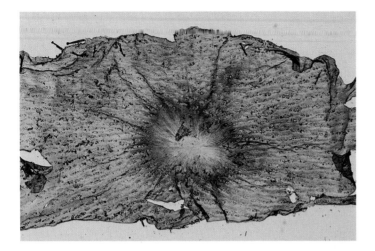

Figure 2.7

Guinea pig skin epidermal sheet (dopa stain) – 1 month after 15 s liquid nitrogen spray. Central melanocytic and pigment loss is seen with epidermal hyperpigmentation at the margins.

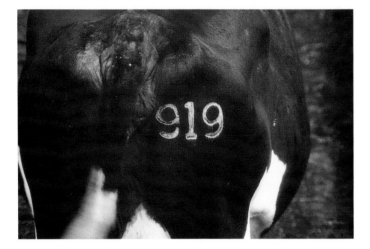

Figure 2.8

Freeze-branded cow showing loss of pigmentation and absence of connective tissue distortion (shape of numbers maintained).

Macroscopic changes

During and immediately after a substantial 30–40 seconds freeze the skin shows a white icefield. Within a few minutes of thawing a violet colour appears at the periphery and moves centrally. Both on the skin and deeper it is clearly demarcated from the surrounding healthy skin. Before long the deeper tissue becomes paler, while a haemorrhagic blister forms on the surface. This turns into an eschar and lasts for a few weeks. The frozen area contracts at 10–14 days.

Microscopic changes

There is essentially no difference between the change seen after cryoprobe or cryospray

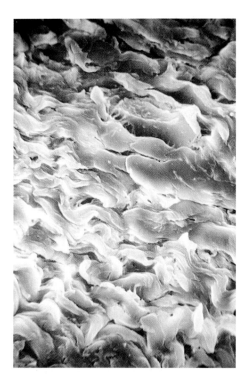

Figure 2.9

Normal upper dermal connective-tissue network (horizontal section) 6 weeks after 25 s liquid nitrogen spray (scanning electron micrograph) ($\times$ 1512.5).

therapy. Ice crystals are seen immediately but the first cellular changes are delayed to about 30 minutes when the cytoplasm shows increasing eosinophilia. There is also margination of the chromatin and vacuolation. Up to 1 hour after freezing there may be no obvious cell death. Over the next few hours there is homogenization of the cytoplasm and nuclear pyknosis. Electron microscopy additionally shows the degranulation of the endoplasmic reticulum. Histologically, blister formation is seen to occur at the dermoepidermal junction (Figure 2.12).

Mechanisms of cellular injury

Ice formation

Extracellular ice damages cell membranes and may be particularly disruptive to tightly packed cells in solid tumours. Intracellular ice also forms in many cells during freezing and is thought to damage mitochondria and endoplasmic reticulum. It is thought to give rise to cellular death even though many cells look quite normal immediately after thawing.

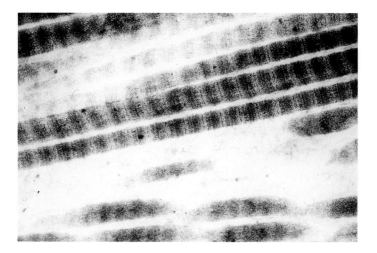

Figure 2.10

Normal collagen fibrils; longitudinal section showing cross-banding pattern of mature fibrils after cryosurgery (transmission electron micrograph).

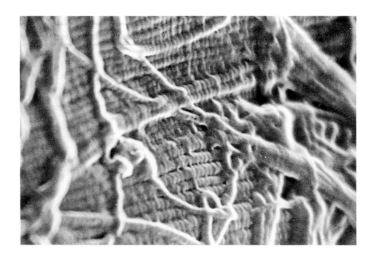

Figure 2.11

Collagen bundle showing individual, normal, cross-banded, collagen fibrils after cryosurgery (scanning electron micrograph) (×96 250).

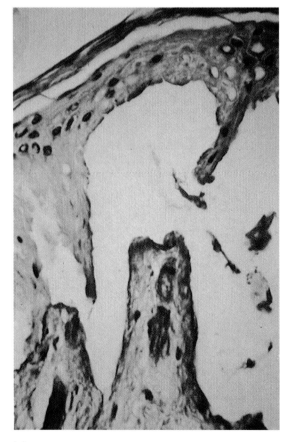

(a)

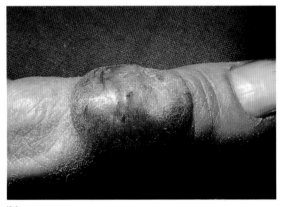

(b)

Figure 2.12

(a) Dermoepidermal split following liquid nitrogen freezing. (Courtesy of Dr D Torre, New York, USA.)

(b) Blister at dermoepidermal junction, following liquid nitrogen spray of a common wart. Bullous Pemphigoid lesions occur at the same depth. Such blisters normally heal without scarring.

Large ice crystals are more damaging than small ones. Slow thawing is associated with recrystallization of ice and this approach is known to be more destructive than rapid thawing.

Osmolarity changes

Extracellular ice is associated with a decrease in extracellular water and an increase in solute concentrations. A change in osmotic gradients leads to a passage of solutes out of cells with a decrease in cellular volume and disruption of cell membranes. Some of the damage is irreversible and the problems are compounded during the reverse process in thawing.

Vascular changes

Flow through capillaries diminishes with modest cold and this is seen readily on the hand in winter when the skin turns white. The effect is less marked in arterioles. Experimentally after liquid nitrogen the first change is vasoconstriction but within 45 minutes of deep freeze vasodilatation supervenes. Showers of microthrombi pass through the capillaries and arterioles and gradually become fixed to the endothelium so that eventually there is no flow at all. This effect can be seen with temperatures of −15°C and below. The result is an ischaemic necrosis which starts around the vessels; its extent will depend on the depth of freeze and its lateral spread. Venules and capillaries are more consistently occluded by the cooling achieved in clinical practice; the vascular necrosis resulting is often therefore a type of 'venous gangrene'. Major arteries are only rarely blocked by freezing of this type.

As with other destructive effects of cryosurgery these vascular changes are more marked after a rapid freeze, slow thaw and refreeze.

Immunology

Much interest has centred on the idea that liquid nitrogen therapy might stimulate the host immune system. It stems from three observations. The first is that, on occasions, treating part of a large wart leads to the disappearance of the whole wart. Secondly, treating one or two viral warts may lead to the resolution of other distant lesions. Thirdly, cryosurgery of a primary tumour has occasionally been associated with the disappearance of distant metastases.

There is some evidence that low temperatures can induce an effective immune recognition of remaining viral or tumour cells. When cells are damaged or killed by freezing they release enzymes, peptides, cytoplasmic components and so on. Some of these may act as antigens and be taken up by antigen presenting cells and presented to lymphocytes. Alternatively, the damaged cells may reveal new antigens on their cell surface. In either case a clone of specific lymphocytes would be induced with the capability of destroying distant virally infected or tumour cells.

Monitoring methods (physical)

Monitoring equipment allows temperature measurements to be made at various distances (vertical and horizontal) from the point of application of the cryogen. Only in this way has it been possible to discover the relationship between depth and dose which is so vital to the science of cryosurgery. Monitoring equipment also has a place in clinical practice. However, with sufficient clinical experience it is often possible to predict the lethality of a cryosurgical dose without monitoring on each occasion. The companies that manufacture cryosurgical equipment either make their own devices or promote compatible monitoring systems.

Instruments useful for monitoring temperature fall into two main groups:

- Thermocouple/pyrometer systems. The meter must read down to about –70°C. It is attached to a thermocouple which is normally housed in a hypodermic needle. The needle is then inserted into the skin, under the tumour if possible; of course, the precise depth of the tumour is not known. However, by use of a slanted jig it is possible to place the needle tip at a predicted depth. One possible error here is if the thermocouple records temperatures conducted down the shaft of the needle.

- Impedance/resistance systems. Electrical impedance in cells increases rapidly when the temperature falls to –40°C. With one electrode positioned in the tumour and the other at a distant point it seems that the flow of a small electric current ceases when the temperature around the tumour electrode falls to about –40°C.

See also Chapter 3.

Bibliography

Arnott J (1851), *On the treatment of cancer by the regulated application of an anaesthetic temperature* (London, J Churchill).

Breitbart EW, Dachów-Siwiéc E (1990), Scientific basis. In: *Advances in cryosurgery: Clinics in dermatology*, ed. Breitbart EW, Dachów-Siwiéc E (New York, Elsevier) Vol 8(1), pp 5–47.

Brodthagen H (1961), Local freezing of the skin by carbon dioxide snow, *Acta Derm-Venereol* (Stockholm) 41 (suppl. 44).

Cooper IS (1963), A new method of destruction or expiration of benign or malignant tumours, *New Engl J Med* 268:743–749.

Cranston Low R (1911), *Carbonic-acid snow as a therapeutic agent in the treatment of disease of the skin* (Edinburgh/London, William Green and Sons).

Dawber RPR (1988), Cold kills! *Clin Exp Dermatol* 13:137–150.

Grimmett R (1961), Liquid nitrogen therapy. Histologic observations, *Arch Dermatol* 83:563–567.

Hall-Edwards J (1913), *Carbon dioxide snow: its therapeutic uses* (London, Simpkin, Marshall, Hamilton, Kent and Co).

Lortat-Jacobs L, Solente G (1930), *La cryothérapie* (Paris, Masson et Cie).

Pusey W (1907), The use of carbon dioxide snow in the treatment of naevi and other lesions of the skin, *JAMA* 49:1354–1356.

Shepherd JP, Dawber RPR (1982), Cryosurgery: History and scientific basis, *Clin Exp Dermatol* 7:321–328.

Torre D (1967), New York, cradle of cryosurgery, *N York State J Med* 67:465–467.

Tytus J (1968), Cryosurgery, its history and development. In: *Cryosurgery*, ed. Rand R, Rinfret A, von Leden H (Springfield, IL, Chas C Thompas) pp 3–18.

White AC (1901), Possibilities of liquid air to the physician, *JAMA* 36:426–428.

Whitehouse H (1907), Liquid air in dermatology: its indications and limitations, *JAMA* 49:371–377.

Zacarian S (1985), Cryogenics: the cryolesion and the pathogenesis of cryonecrosis. In: *Cryosurgery for skin cancer and cutaneous disorders*, ed. Zacarian SA (St Louis, Mosby Co) pp 1–30.

3 Equipment and techniques

During the last 25 years liquid nitrogen has increasingly superseded all other refrigerants for use in dermatological cryosurgery. This is reflected in the equipment that has evolved and the techniques that are now used in routine office practice. In this section particular attention is therefore given to methods using liquid nitrogen. Details of other types of apparatus still used in some parts of the world can be obtained from the references at the end of this chapter.

Cryosurgery does not involve the removal of tissue and its techniques are not as exactly reproducible as excisional surgery or radiotherapy. It is therefore very important to have a good understanding of the equipment and techniques that are involved. Complex methods should not be attempted until simple ones have been mastered; also standardization of whatever procedure is adopted is crucial. The precise treatment given can then be documented and if necessary an enhanced treatment can be given should the initial regimen fail to cure. It is also important to learn that different lesions will have varying sensitivity to cold.

Liquid nitrogen supply and storage

In most countries the manufacturers and suppliers of cryosurgery equipment also produce liquid nitrogen storage devices or provide the names of companies who market them and supply liquid nitrogen. With regard to the latter it is important to state that any medical practitioner wishing to carry out simple cryosurgery to lesions such as warts and benign keratoses may be able to obtain a supply of liquid nitrogen from a variety of sources—it is extensively used all over the world in universities, hospitals and most engineering and electrical research units. Such departments are usually willing to supply small amounts of liquid nitrogen for clinical use. Under these circumstances one only requires a vacuum flask of adequate size with a hole punctured through the lid. A standard 1–2 litre vacuum flask may be adequate but if regular treatment sessions are to be undertaken a metal vacuum container specifically designed for refrigerant storage is desirable.

These are robust and last for many years without vacuum failure occurring.

Since liquid nitrogen boils at –196°C and will explode if retained in a totally sealed container, the storage vessels are designed to allow some degree of leakage or evaporation. In order to maintain adequate supplies of liquid nitrogen for regular clinical use it is important to note storage capacity in relation to evaporation rates (Table 3.1).

The agitation generated by decanting the liquid into the treatment equipment leads to considerable wastage. To avoid this many storage flasks can be fitted with pressure head withdrawal devices which dispense the liquid nitrogen at rates of up to 8–10 litres/min. The cost of such equipment has to be balanced against the expenditure for more frequent liquid nitrogen supplies.

Table 3.1 Vacuum container capacities and holding times.

Storage capacity (litres)	Static holding time (days)
5	6
10	45
25	110
35	110
50	125

Liquid nitrogen spray and probes

In routine clinical practice, liquid nitrogen spray equipment has become increasingly dominant over other methods—the equipment is convenient and very easy to use and essentially similar methods can be used for benign, premalignant and malignant lesions—giving success rates at least on a par with irradiation and excisional surgery, but without the complexity of these treatment modalities.

The most popular units used in office practice are basically small, metal or plastic vacuum flasks with a screw-on top possessing a spray-release system and a valve giving a working pressure of 6 psi (41.4 kPa) and safety relief pressure of approximately 70 psi (483 kPa) (Figure 3.1). The liquid nitrogen capacity of the most frequently used units is no more than 500 ml. The various spray attachments on the unit head are either screw-on or have a LeurLock fitting as for syringe needles. The most widely used units (Brymill Corporation cryospray range) have a range of four screw-on brass spray tips with diameters from 1 mm down to 0.375 mm, labelled A to D respectively. In general, sprays B and C are preferred, as they give sufficient concentration and scatter of liquid nitrogen for treating skin lesions, particularly when the 'spot-freeze' method is employed. Spray tip A, used at 1 cm distance from the skin surface, can be seen to cause liquid nitrogen to bounce off the skin and be scattered over several centimetres, giving greater inflammatory morbidity. It should be reserved for the treatment of large malignant lesions.

Spray technique

For other than benign, regular lesions, the field to be treated is delineated with a skin marker pen. For most benign lesions this will

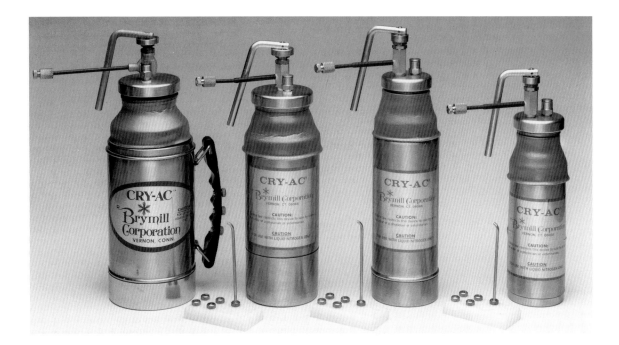

Figure 3.1

Stages in the development of the CRY-AC handheld liquid nitrogen spray/probe equipment: (from left to right) original strap handle (1975); current model (1983); new model (1989); CRY-AC-3 (1989) (Brymill Corporation, USA).

be approximately 1–2 mm beyond the visible pathological margin; for premalignant and malignant lesions a margin of up to 1 cm of clinically normal skin may be included. The directional spray method employed to treat lesions of differing sizes may be the spot-freeze, paint-spray, rotatory or spiral technique (Figure 3.2)—in the UK the spot-freeze method is most frequently used.

In this latter method the liquid nitrogen spray tip is held approximately 1 cm from the skin over the centre of the area to be treated. If the distance from the tip of the spray to the skin surface requires exact standardization, the authors use plastic jigs for this purpose. Spraying is commenced and the white ice spreads outwards forming a circular 'icefield'.

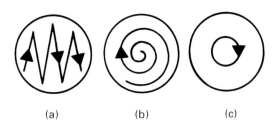

(a)   (b)   (c)

Figure 3.2

Various liquid nitrogen spray directional techniques used to provide *even* ice production within the defined treatment field: (**a**) paint-brush, (**b**) spiral and (**c**) rotary.

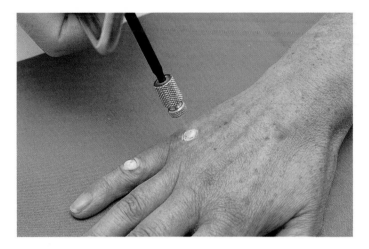

Figure 3.3

Cryosurgery to several hand warts.

When ice has developed within the desired field the spray is maintained with sufficient pressure to keep the field frozen for the length of time considered adequate—from 5 to 30 seconds depending on the pathology of the lesion; more than 30 seconds may be required occasionally but this can induce connective tissue disruption and scarring (see Chapter 7). The spot-freeze method is only satisfactory for fields of up to 2 cm diameter (Figure 3.3); beyond this size, the temperature of any ice seen to form is greater than –15°C and therefore not low enough to give adequate cell killing: edge recurrences (or persistence) may develop whatever the nature of the lesion.

If the lesion to be treated by the spot-freeze method is greater than 2 cm diameter then the 'field' is divided into overlapping circles of 2 cm diameter that are each treated separately. Alternatively, the paint-spray or spiral spray technique may be used, ensuring an even spray and depth of freeze across the whole lesion.

The appropriate freeze regime is employed depending on the nature of the lesion, and recorded in the treatment notes, for example, as follows:

Note: LN$_2$ Single icefield 1 × 5 seconds

Meaning: Liquid nitrogen Lesion <2 cm: frozen once for 5 seconds after ice formed in the defined field.

The spot-freeze method was developed in an attempt to standardize cryosurgery treatment so that:

- Medical personnel of limited experience could use the method in exactly the same way, and obtain the same success rates, as more experienced practitioners;
- Accurate knowledge could be obtained regarding the relative sensitivity or resistance of different lesions to cryosurgery;
- If treatment should fail, then one could exactly repeat, or lengthen, the second spray.

The techniques involved in various centres to define the adequacy of 'icefield' formation and satisfactory cell killing vary considerably, particularly with regard to assessing the depth of freeze. It is generally agreed that the lateral spread of ice is the most practical method of

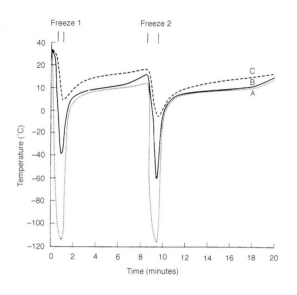

Figure 3.4

Temperatures recorded during two freeze–thaw cycles of liquid nitrogen spray (30 s after icefield formation) **(A)** at 2 mm depth, **(B)** 6 mm depth and **(C)** 10 mm depth.

judging depth. Using the spot-freeze method for each 2 cm circle treated, the maximum depth of adequate ice formation in the centre of the lesion will be at least 0.5 cm (i.e. a 4:1 ratio). That adequate 'killing' temperatures are obtained within this field has been confirmed by animal-model studies (i.e. temperatures lower than −40°C occur within this field) (Figure 3.4).

Probe technique

All the commercially available handheld and benchbased machines with spray attachments also have a variety of metal probes through which liquid nitrogen is circulated to cool the tip which is to be applied to the lesion. These vary in size and are usually circular—from 1 mm up to several centimetres in diameter (Figure 3.5). In order to obtain adequate skin contact with the cooled probe, the probe is dried before freezing and lubricant jelly applied to the skin. A probe is selected of a size equivalent to the field to be treated. The probe is placed on the lesion and cooling is commenced.

The probe adheres to the lubricant jelly and skin within 5–6 seconds. It is then gently retracted from the skin, thereby protecting surrounding tissues from unnecessary freezing and inflammation. The treatment is then continued for from 10 seconds to 2 minutes depending on the diameter and pathology of the treatment field. The probe cannot immediately be removed at this stage because of the iceball effect between the skin and probe—allow between 10 and 30 seconds for sufficient thawing to permit separation to occur.

Many other spray and probe techniques have been described which are detailed in the bibliography; it is most important, however, to gain experience with one method by:

- Experimenting with animal tissue such as pig feet or hock available from most meat retailers (Figure 3.6);
- Reading the experience gained by others in the past on models such as the pig flank;
- Observing experienced operators—this is particularly valuable with regard to malignant lesions since much of the therapeutic failure can be ascribed to poor technique.

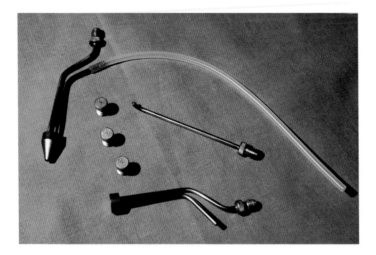

Figure 3.5

Screw-in attachments for the CRY-AC liquid nitrogen handheld unit. Metal probes through which the liquid nitrogen is circulated are to the left and below (Brymill Corporation, USA).

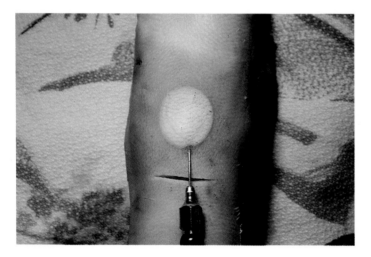

Figure 3.6

Pig's foot and hock as used in dermatological surgery workshops here being used to demonstrate the thermocouple depth dose monitor in situ below the frozen icefield.

If a second freeze is required, as it is with most malignant tumours, then complete thawing is important after the initial freeze. With liquid nitrogen equipment this can be judged as the time at which the ice has disappeared and can no longer be felt on palpation. This stage is usually more than 3–4 times the duration of the freeze time after ice formation. Much cellular injury occurs during the thaw phase and complete, as opposed to partial, thawing decreases cell survival.

The liquid nitrogen equipment and methods described above are as used with handheld devices. The more complex and larger benchbased units involve exactly the same principles for clinical practice; many have built-in monitoring facilities which are only needed to treat larger, malignant lesions.

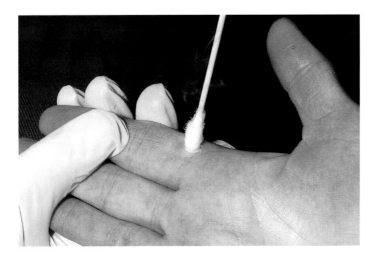

Figure 3.7

Cotton-wool bud application of liquid nitrogen. The ice formed can be seen extending on to normal skin by about 1 mm.

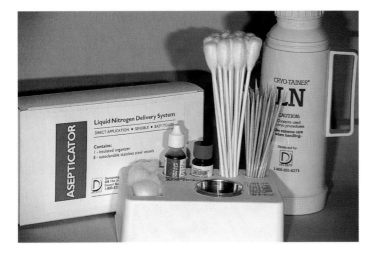

Figure 3.8

Liquid nitrogen (cotton-wool bud) delivery system (Delasco) designed to avoid viral cross-contamination between patients.

Cotton-wool bud technique

This is the simplest method of applying liquid nitrogen to skin lesions. Although largely superseded by liquid nitrogen cryospray, the technique is still quite widely used in hospital dermatology outpatient clinics and in primary care for the treatment of warts and thin keratosis.

The treatment process involves dipping the cotton-wool bud into the liquid nitrogen and firmly applying it to the lesion until a narrow halo of white ice forms around the bud. This is a useful treatment endpoint which occurs within seconds. For larger lesions, redipping and re-application of the bud may be necessary; the duration of each application will depend on the size and

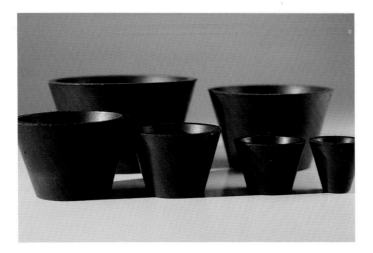

Figure 3.9

Neoprene cones used to concentrate liquid nitrogen spray and limit its lateral spread.

nature of the lesion to be treated (Figure 3.7).

When using the cotton-wool bud technique, the area of the tip of cotton wool should be slightly smaller than the area to be treated. The liquid nitrogen should first be decanted into a small metal gallipot placed within another open container, ensuring easy access and less spillage. This also protects the main liquid nitrogen supply from the risk of cross-contamination with viruses such as human papilloma virus, herpes virus and hepatitis strains which can remain viable at temperatures as low as –196°C. For this reason some manufacturers such as Delasco (Frigiderm Asepticator System) have designed cheap equipment to individualize the cotton-bud method (Figure 3.8).

It is not possible to standardize the cotton-wool method due to many variables—the ambient temperature, the pressure applied, the distance the bud travels between the liquid nitrogen and the lesion and 'dripping' of the liquid. One cannot obtain temperatures lower than –20°C below a depth of 2–3 mm with this technique; it is therefore only suitable for treating relatively small, superficial benign skin lesions.

Other equipment

When using the liquid nitrogen spray technique, various standard pieces of equipment or objects used in an improvised manner, may be used to localise the area of spray or to protect the surrounding tissue.

Truncated neoprene, nonconducting cones (Figure 3.9)

These are frequently used to concentrate the spray and limit its lateral spread. A cone of sufficient size is chosen to encompass the field to be frozen. The completion of treatment is judged as the time at which a 1–2 mm halo of ice forms outside the cone after continuous liquid nitrogen spray inside the cone. Auroscope earpieces may be used instead for smaller lesions.

The cone spray technique gives a very rapid rate of temperature decrease which is probably more destructive than the open spray method. It also limits the lateral spread of spray and ice; this can be useful at sites such as the eyelids and inner canthus. Some modern machines have an attachable 'closed

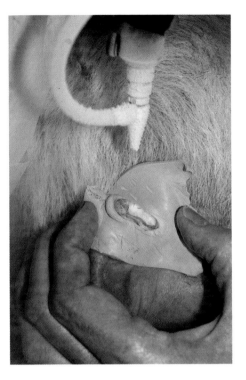

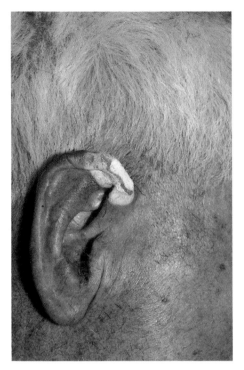

Figure 3.10

(a) Adhesive putty – an appropriately sized piece has been chosen to surround the field to be treated on the ear.

(b) Icefield induced – putty removed.

cone' which is pressed on to the skin and into which the liquid nitrogen is sprayed.

Eye protectors

When periocular lesions are to be treated the orbit of the eye can be protected by a plastic eye-protector; a smooth edged plastic spoon may suffice. When spraying the lower eyelid a Jaeger eyelid retractor may be particularly useful.

Adhesive putty

Adhesive putty (Figure 3.10) is normally used for sticking objects such as posters on walls. It can be used in cryosurgery to treat large or irregular lesions or those adjacent to vital structures such as the eye. The edge of the lesion is first defined with a marker pen, including a margin of clinically normal skin when required. An appropriately sized piece of adhesive putty is then applied to surround the field to be treated. When the liquid nitrogen spray is carried out, the putty freezes to the circumscribed skin, thus protecting the normal surrounding skin from freeze injury. Because freezing occurs slightly beyond the putty margin, a less rigid margin of pigment change is seen after healing, thus giving a better cosmetic result than that produced by the cone spray method.

Monitoring equipment

In our experience monitoring equipment which measures either adequacy of the ice formation or temperature is quite unnecessary in routine practice—if only benign lesions and small or superficial malignancies are to be treated. To understand the cryobiological justification for this statement the reader is referred to the detailed references at the end of this chapter and of Chapter 2. For larger tumours 'depth dose' monitoring is probably useful and generally considered necessary. The reservation is based on the premiss that no physical method can guarantee to measure adequate cell death.

Most machines involve the use of thermocouple/pyrometer technology and impedance/resistance methods; experimental techniques include heat flowmetrics and thermography.

Other refrigerants

With the worldwide availability of liquid nitrogen sprays and probes, carbon dioxide snow methodology has become somewhat obsolete. However, if only carbon dioxide snow-making equipment is available it is capable of giving good results for most benign lesions and small superficial basal cell carcinomas.

Nitrous oxide cooled (Joule–Thomson effect) probes are widely used for internal lesions in gynaecology, oral surgery and ophthalmology. In practice they have limited value in dermatology, mainly because of the availability, simplicity and greater efficacy of liquid nitrogen machines. The practical techniques used for surface freezing with nitrous oxide probes are similar to those carried out with liquid nitrogen probes.

Fluorocarbon liquids

Fluorocarbon liquids (e.g. dichlorodifluoromethane) can be used in the spray mode and are produced commercially in siphon cans with extension nozzles. It is possible to obtain surface temperatures as low as –60°C with some of these units but with very little depth penetration; they may have valves allowing for fine, medium and coarse spraying. They are suitable for broad-based superficial field treatment (e.g. diffuse acne comedones or pitted scars).

The Histofreezer (Thames Laboratories, UK) is sold as a convenient, easy to use, aerosol for the treatment of warts. It consists of a kit containing a 150 ml dimethyl-ether-propane aerosol with 40 cotton-bud applicators; the latter can apparently be cooled down to –50°C for use on warts. The cell-killing effect of this method is likely to be considerably less efficient than the cotton-bud liquid nitrogen regimen. Using needle probe equipment to measure skin temperatures (up to 1 mm deep) we were not able to detect tissue temperatures much below 0°C—evidently this method needs considerably more objective clinical studies to assess its possible efficacy.

Bibliography

Colver GB, Dawber RPR (1991), Malignant spots: spot freezes. In: *Surgical gems in dermatology*, ed. Robins P (New York/Tokyo, Igaku-Shoin) Vol 2, pp 1417.

Torre D (1990), Cryosurgical instrumentation and depth dose monitoring. In: *Advances in cryosurgery: Clinics in dermatology*, ed. Breitbart EW, Dachów-Siwiéc E (New York, Elsevier) Vol 8(1), pp 4859.

Torre D, Lubritz R, Kuflik E (1988), Practical cutaneous cryosurgery (Norwalk, CT, Appleton & Lange).

4 Benign lesions

This chapter deals with the heart of cryosurgery—the rapid and effective treatment of common benign skin lesions.

How effective is cryosurgery?

When dealing with the benign lesions discussed in this chapter dermatologists would regard cryosurgery as the mainstay of treatment for viral warts and seborrhoeic keratoses. High cure rates and low morbidity can be expected. Indeed with thin seborrhoeic warts success is virtually guaranteed. For viral warts it is wise to be cautiously optimistic because sometimes even innocuous-looking warts can prove very resistant to therapy.

The other tumours and diseases listed in this chapter will all be suitable for cryosurgery in some situations but not others. It is very important to realize that cure is not certain and repeated or aggressive freezing of resistant lesions should be avoided.

Principles of treatment

Most epidermal, warty lesions are easy to recognize and amenable to cryosurgery. Deep freezing is unnecessary and will produce side-effects. Keratin is an excellent insulator so when dealing with a thick lesion it may be difficult to achieve subzero temperatures at the base. The keratin can be debulked with a curette or scalpel prior to freezing. Seborrhoeic keratoses seem to sit on the skin and a good result is possible with very little inflammation of surrounding or deep tissue. Some viral warts, however, depending on the subtype of human papilloma virus producing the lesion, have a deeper component and considerable swelling and tissue destruction may accompany successful treatment.

In some individuals blistering is seen after short and superficial freezes, whereas others may tolerate more prolonged or deeper freezes with only minimal oedema. It is prudent therefore to freeze cautiously at the first visit and to record accurately, in the patient's notes, the duration of freeze (see under techniques in Chapter 3). A suitable freeze at the first visit would be a single 5 second freeze–thaw cycle.

When the diagnosis is in doubt a biopsy should be taken. Remember that warty thickening can be a feature of premalignant and malignant tumours.

Patient information

Cryosurgery can be a puzzling and painful experience for patients. The concept of burning off a wart with a cold liquid is 'foreign' and the steaming vacuum flask or complex equipment does nothing to reassure them. Occasionally someone will faint from the concern and discomfort of the procedure. It is therefore important not to pounce with cotton-wool bud or spray in hand, but first to explain calmly what will happen. The information must cover the procedure but also the after-effects. It is wise to give written instructions because most people forget what they are told in the heat of the moment. Table 4.1 gives details of a suggested information leaflet for cryosurgery of benign epidermal lesions. Each physician will want to vary it according to local factors.

Table 4.1   **Advice sheet following cryosurgery for benign lesions.**

PATIENT INFORMATION LEAFLET CRYOSURGERY

Your wart/verruca/skin lump has been treated with liquid nitrogen. The wart is destroyed by freezing it to a temperature well below zero. Some stinging starts during treatment, and may continue through thawing, but settles within a few minutes. If you get pain later on take 1 or 2 paracetamol (acetaminophen) tablets.

Redness and some swelling can be expected. In a day or two a water (or blood) blister may form, especially where the skin is thin and sensitive. A small blister should be covered with an adhesive dressing. If you get a large blister simply let out the fluid with a sterile, pointed instrument; repeat this until the blister no longer refills and apply an antiseptic cream twice daily.

The wart, or part of it, may peel or drop off in a week or two and a further scaly crust may form on the wound.

If you have any cause for concern please contact the surgery for advice. Remember that you may require further treatment in 3 or 4 weeks.

Viral warts

Viral warts are common and affect between 5 and 10 per cent of all children at any one time. The peak incidence is in the early teenage years. Several subtypes of human papilloma virus produce different morphological varieties of wart.

Approximately 65 per cent of warts disappear spontaneously within 2 years. The figure is probably higher for plantar warts, especially those occurring in children.

Common warts

These may appear anywhere but are usually seen on the face, hands and knees (Figures 4.1–4.3). Size may range from a millimetre to over a centimetre. They have a rough surface and the epidermal ridges do not cross the wart. There are rarely any symptoms but occasionally a wart may bleed readily and be sore. The diagnosis is usually clear to the doctor and patient (Figure 4.4).

Plane warts

These are smooth, flat-topped papules and may occur in large numbers on the face or back of the hands. The colour may be pale, pink or brown. They range roughly from 1 to 5 mm in diameter (Figures 4.5, 4.6). Some are so small that they can only be seen properly with side-lighting. They may persist for years and be cosmetically embarrassing but here cryosurgery must be carefully considered. The large number of lesions and the risk of pigmentary change may persuade the doctor to avoid freezing.

Plantar warts (verrucas)

The rough surface may protrude only slightly from the skin and there may be a surrounding horny collar. These lesions may be

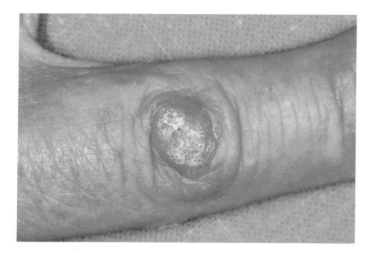

Figure 4.1

Viral wart over the proximal, inter-phalangeal joint.

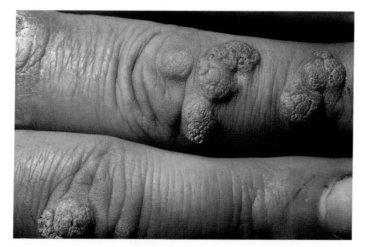

Figure 4.2

Multiple (common) viral warts.

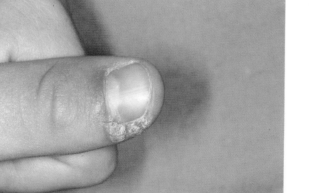

Figure 4.3

Periungual warts – care is needed at this site to avoid treatment causing nail matrix atrophy and permanent scarring.

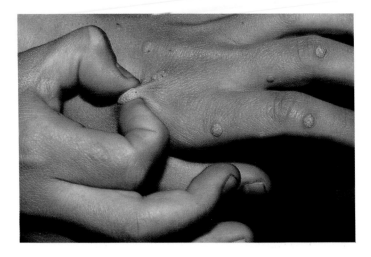

Figure 4.4

This boy diagnosed his own warts –
here he is demonstrating his own
method of attempted removal!

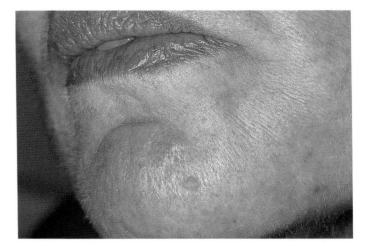

Figure 4.5

Solitary brown plane wart on the
chin.

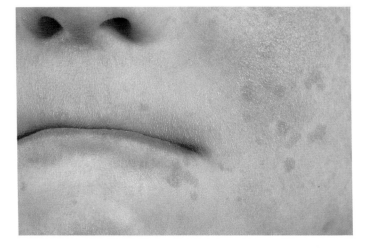

Figure 4.6

Numerous orange-brown plane warts
on the cheek.

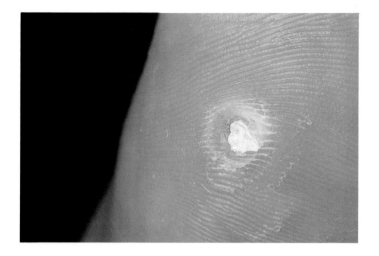

Figure 4.7

(a) Verruca with surface maceration and oedema following treatment with a salicylic acid plaster.

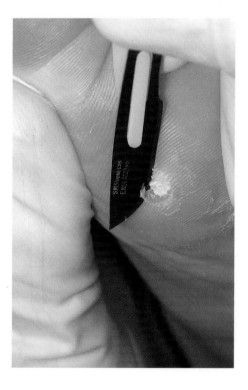

(b) Paring down the keratin.

painful, particularly if the keratin builds up. When pared down capillary bleeding may be seen. Epidermal ridges do not cross the verruca and this helps to distinguish them from corns. Mosaic warts are made up of multiple small individual lesions and they may be several centimetres in diameter (Figure 4.7).

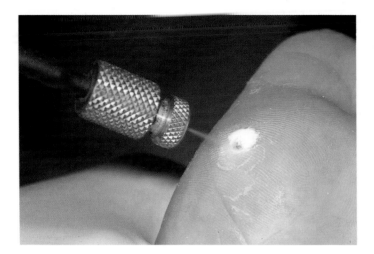

Figure 4.7 *(continued)*
(**c**) Cryosurgery (liquid nitrogen spray) in action.

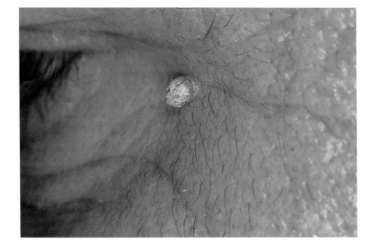

Figure 4.8
Digitate wart.

Filiform or digitate warts

These finger or frondlike warts are more common in men on the face, neck and scalp (Figures 4.8, 4.9).

Anogenital warts

These are not described here because it is necessary to investigate for other sexually transmitted diseases and this should be done by an appropriate specialist.

Treatment

For common and plantar warts home treatment is most appropriate. A salicylic acid-containing wart preparation should be used for up to 12 weeks (Figure 4.10). This applies

to continue the good work; when, a week or so after freezing, the redness and swelling settle the patient should use an emery board each night prior to applying a wart paint.

Cryosurgical technique

In older children and adults it is often justifiable to freeze warts.

It is wise to start conservatively and to document the time. If at the next visit there has been little reaction the freezing time can be increased accordingly. The cryospray is very convenient. A 1 mm halo ring should be allowed to form on the normal skin surrounding the wart; multiple warts can be treated quickly in this way (Figure 4.11). Pinpoint accuracy can be achieved, if necessary, by spraying down a small auroscope earpiece or neoprene cone which is placed over the wart (Figure 4.12).

With the dipstick technique a cotton-wool bud, slightly smaller than the wart, is used. It is dipped into liquid nitrogen and applied firmly and vertically on to the wart (Figure 4.13). A halo 1 mm wide should be allowed to form on the normal skin around the base of the wart. This may take 2 or 3 seconds for a small wart, but up to 30 seconds for a large one. Once the icefield is established it should be maintained for about 5 seconds at the first treatment. It is more difficult to assess the time required for a plantar wart because it is not raised and the 1 mm halo rule is less reliable; it is usually 10–30 seconds.

Filiform warts need a different approach. It may be difficult to position the patient such that a wart under the chin is downhill from the nitrogen source. Cotton-wool buds are not very practical at this site, but a spray can be directed sideways at the lesion. Alternatively an angled spray adaptor is available on some models to direct the spray upwards.

Cryosurgery produces swelling and a ring on the finger may become impossible to

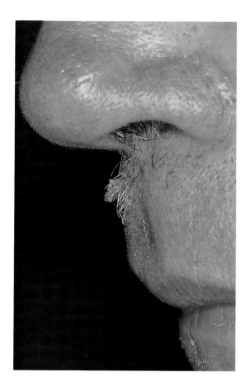

Figure 4.9

Digitate wart.

particularly to young children. Cryosurgery is painful and it is not always appropriate to inflict it on unsuspecting youngsters as first-line treatment. However, the application of a local anaesthetic cream (e.g. EMLA: Astra Pharm) 1–2 hours prior to therapy may be useful if treatment is to be considered. Keratin is such a good insulator that the freezing of markedly hyperkeratotic lesions is less successful. They can be pared down before freezing, but the patient must be encouraged

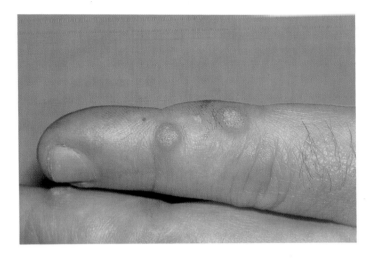

Figure 4.10

(a) Home treatment of a viral wart.

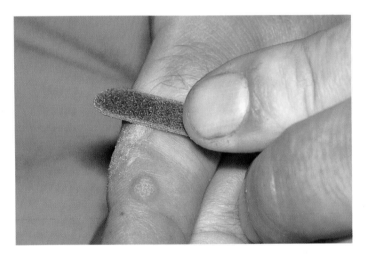

(b) Keratin is abraded with an emery board.

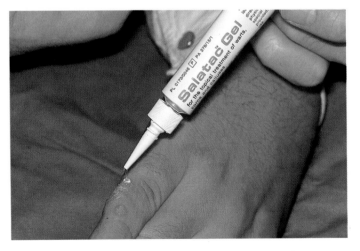

(c) A salicylic acid containing collodion is applied.

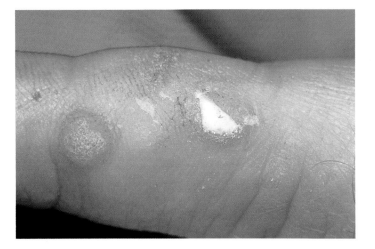

(**d**) Within a few minutes the collodion dries. This can be repeated each night for several weeks.

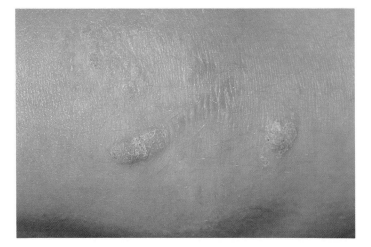

Figure 4.11

(**a**) Several warts arising in scars on both knees.

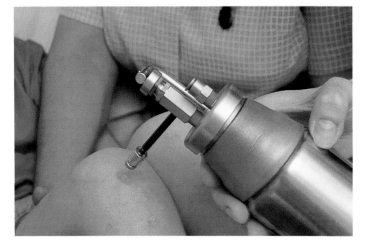

(**b**) Cryosurgery is a rapid method of treatment.

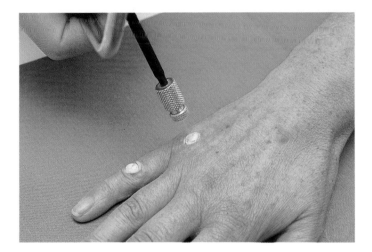

Figure 4.11 *(continued)*

(**c**) Cryosurgery to several hand warts.

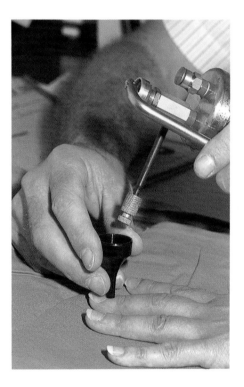

Figure 4.12

Auroscope earpieces are available in several sizes and can be useful for accurate localization of the liquid nitrogen spray.

remove. It is essential to take off any ring before freezing a lesion on the finger (Figure 4.14).

Maximum success is achieved by treating the warts at approximately 3-weekly intervals. Treatment intervals longer than 6 weeks lower the cure rate and treating more frequently may not give time for the previous inflammation to settle down. It is wise to get an impetus going with regular visits and to ask the patient to revert to a wart paint between visits. In this manner nearly 85 per cent of warts can be cleared in 12 weeks. In fact this figure is little better than using a wart paint alone but many wart paint failures will respond to cryosurgery.

Molluscum contagiosum

This is another common viral infection (synonym: 'water warts'; Figure 4.15). Children are chiefly affected, particularly those with atopic eczema. The number of lesions

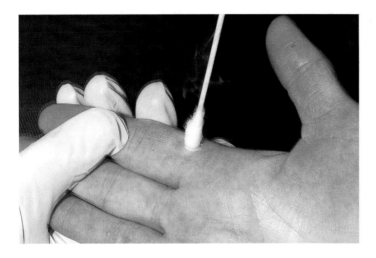

Figure 4.13
Cotton-wool bud application of liquid nitrogen. The ice formed can be seen extending on to normal skin by about 1 mm.

present may vary from one or two to several hundreds and they can persist for months or years. Several techniques have been described which are effective in dealing with these lesions. A sharpened orange stick steeped in phenol can be inserted into the surface. Each lesion can be squeezed with forceps until some cheesy matter appears. Neither of these methods is readily accepted by young children and it may therefore be best to apply a wart paint, as for common warts. Alternatively, after the child soaks in a warm bath for 10 minutes, the surface of each molluscum can be rubbed gently with a pumice stone.

Cryosurgical technique

This can rarely be used for children under the age of 6 years without the prior application of EMLA cream two hours before treatment. Either a cotton-wool bud dipped in nitrogen or a spray gun can be used. Nitrogen is applied until the surface of the lesion is white. This

takes a few seconds. The central dimple, so characteristic of molluscum, is highlighted. It is not necessary to freeze until a 1 mm halo appears on the surrounding skin. Over the next few days there may be temporary swelling then shrinkage and the papule falls off. Secondary bacterial infection is not uncommon and it may therefore be necessary to prescribe a topical antibiotic concurrently.

Seborrhoeic warts (keratoses)

These benign tumours are common in Caucasians and are often accepted as a normal change of ageing. They become more common after 50 years of age, but may even be seen in the third decade. Single lesions occur but they may be multiple and sometimes familial.

The clinical features are variable (Figures 4.16–4.21). The most common appearance is a rough surfaced plaque apparently stuck on the skin surface. Other features are listed in Table 4.2.

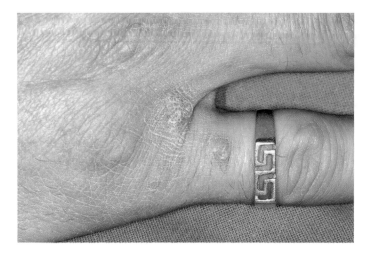

Figure 4.14

(a) It is essential to remove rings from a finger before cryosurgery.

(b) The ring has been removed and the wart is frozen.

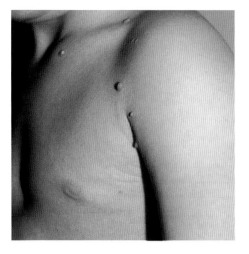

Figure 4.15

Molluscum contagiosum lesions are often multiple.

Table 4.2 Features of seborrhoeic warts.

Colour:	Grey, yellow, brown or black, but may be varied (Figures 4.16 and 4.17)
Size:	From 1 mm to many centimetres (Figures 4.18 and 4.19)
Distribution:	Face, central trunk common; hair-bearing skin possible
Surface:	Usually rough or crumbly; dull; may resemble 'currant bun'; occasionally may have a shiny surface (Figure 4.20)

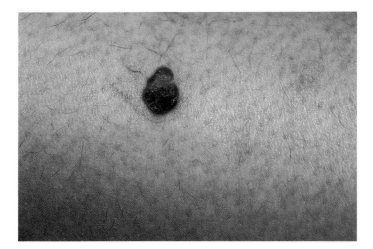

Figure 4.16

Seborrhoeic warts may show variation in colour.

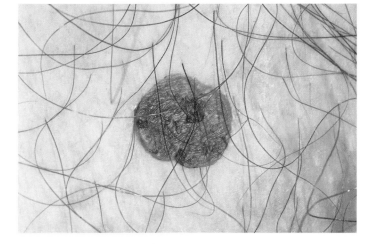

Figure 4.17

Seborrhoeic warts, showing variation in colour—see also Figure 4.16.

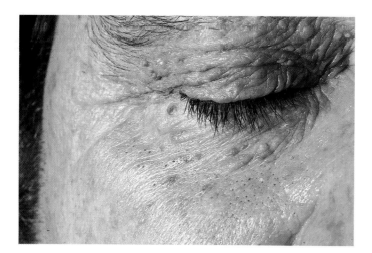

Figure 4.18

Multiple small seborrhoeic warts around the eye.

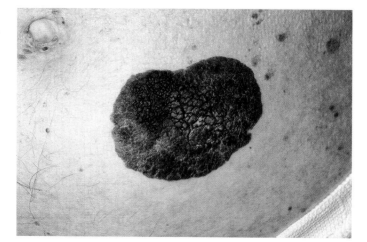

Figure 4.19

Large, dull, rough seborrhoeic warts.

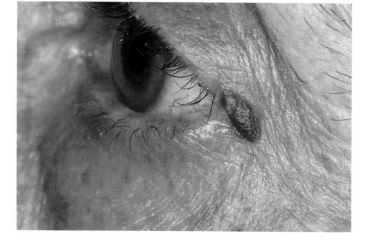

Figure 4.20

Seborrhoeic wart with a shiny surface.

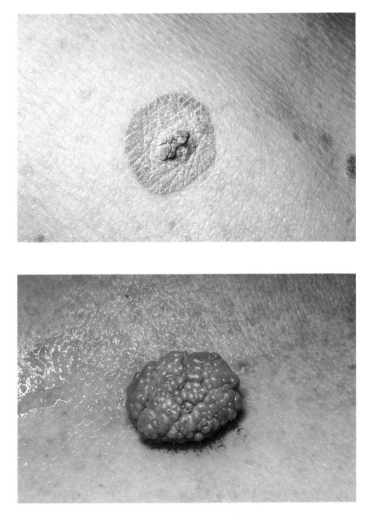

Figure 4.21

Flat seborrhoeic wart with a fine patterned surface. This lesion had recently produced a central, raised keratotic area, making clinical diagnosis easier.

Figure 4.22

Some melanocytic naevi show morphological features similar to seborrhoeic keratoses—this one is 'fleshy' to the touch.

Special varieties

Flat

All seborrhoeic keratoses begin life as flat lesions but most become raised at an early stage. Some, however, extend radially and may reach several centimetres in diameter. They can then be confused with other flat brown lesions, e.g. lentigo maligna and senile lentigo. The keratosis may retain a fine patterned fissured surface as a differentiating feature (Figure 4.21). If in doubt take a biopsy to confirm the diagnosis.

Pedunculated

This type, which grows away from the skin with a narrow neck, is seen particularly in the axillae, inguinal region and on the eyelids.

Some melanocytic naevi are pedunculated and their colour may also vary between pink and black. It may be difficult to differentiate between them but naevi tend to have a fleshy feel (Figure 4.22).

Infected

It is not uncommon for at least one part of a wart to become infected; this may lead to itching, bleeding and concern. On examination there may be swelling, redness, pustulation and the pigment may deepen. A few days of antibiotic cream may resolve the diagnostic dilemma.

When to treat

It is usually for cosmetic reasons that people demand treatment. Friends may have commented that a particular lesion is ugly. Not uncommonly it is a grandchild tugging at a wart, and saying that it is horrid, that persuades a grandparent to visit the doctor. Treatment is easy and it is hard to refuse the request when the wart is patently disfiguring.

Keratoses may catch on garments, causing a nuisance, and may bleed or become inflamed in the process. Itching (sometimes intermittent) may also be a problem.

With increasing publicity about the early detection of skin cancer, more people now attend doctors with pigmented lesions. Fortunately most seborrhoeic warts are readily diagnosed. However, when there is doubt it is best to refer to a specialist or investigate by biopsy or removal.

How to treat

Keratoses are rewarding tumours to treat because they are on a separate level from the surrounding skin and new epidermis covers the wound within 7–10 days. Either curettage or shave excision give excellent cosmetic results and provide a histological specimen. Local anaesthetic is required. These methods are particularly useful for large heaped-up keratoses for which liquid nitrogen is not usually suitable because keratin is such a good insulator.

For standard keratoses, up to a few millimetres thick, or for the pedunculated variety, liquid nitrogen can be used in much the same way as for viral warts. A spot freeze with cotton-wool bud or cryospray is satisfactory—the ice halo should encroach on to normal skin by 1 mm.

If wide (over 1.5 cm) lesions are treated by the spot-freeze method the freeze at the centre will be unnecessarily deep. For this type the 'paint spray technique' can be used (see Figure 3.2): the spray-gun nozzle is slowly moved over the surface of the keratosis to effect an even distribution of freeze. Compared to the spot-freeze method this is less standardized because the element of movement has been introduced, giving less uniform freezing. However, these are not malignant tumours and a margin of error is permissible. With practice it is possible to create a fairly reproducible technique that will successfully remove the majority of seborrhoeic warts without undue morbidity.

Spectrum of amenable lesions (Table 4.3)

Cells vary in their susceptibility to freezing and some, such as melanocytes, are readily destroyed whereas others, such as fibroblasts, are more resistant. It follows that some tumours will be amenable to conservative liquid nitrogen treatment while others will respond only to more aggressive therapy. When dealing with benign tumours it may

Table 4.3 Practical treatment schedules (spot freeze method when sprayed).

Commoner benign lesions Lesion	Technique	Time (secs)	FTC	Margin	Sessions	Interval (weeks)
Acne						
Cyst	P or OS	5–10	1	—	2–3	4
Comedones	Peel	Ice formation	1	—	1	—
Vulgaris (mixed lesions)	Peel	Ice formation	1	—	1	—
Scarring 'Ice pick'	Peel	Ice formation	1	—	1	—
Keloidalis (nape of neck)	P	30	1	—	3	6
Adenoma sebaceum	P	10–15	1	—	3	4–8
Alopecia areata	OS	5	1	—	1	—
Angiokeratoma						
Mibelli	P or OS	10	1	1 mm	3	8
Scrotum	P or OS	10	1	1 mm	3	8
Angiolymphoid hyperplasia	OS	15	1	—	1	—
Cherry angioma	P	10	1	—	1	—
Chondrodermatitis nodularis helicis	OS	15	1	2 mm	3	6
Clear cell acanthoma	OS	20	1	2–3 mm	1	—
Cutaneous horn	OS	10–15	1	2 mm	1	—
Dermatofibroma	P	20	1	2 mm	2	8–10
Dermatosis papulosa nigrans	P or F	5	1	1 mm	1	—
Dissem. superficial actinic keratosis	OS	3–5	1	1 mm	1	—
Elastosis perforans serpiginosa	OS	10	1	1 mm	2	6–8
Epidermal naevus	OS or P	5	1	1 mm	2	6
Granuloma annulare	OS or P	5–10	1	—	2	8
Granuloma faciale	OS or P	5–10	1	—	2	8
Haemangioma	P	20	1	—	2–4	8
Herpes labialis – recurrent	OS	10	1	—	1	—
Hidradenitis suppurativa	OS	15	1	—	2–3	6
Hyperhidrosis – axillary	OS	15	1	—	2	8
Hypertrophic scar	OS or P	20–25	1	2 mm	1	—
Idiopathic guttate melanosis	OS	5	1	—	2	4–6

Table 4.3 continued

Commoner benign lesions Lesion	Technique	Time (secs)	FTC	Margin	Sessions	Interval (weeks)
Ingrowing toenail ·	OS	20	1	2 mm	2	6–8
Keloid	OS or P	30	1	2–3 mm	3	8
Kyrle's disease	OS	10	1	1 mm	1	—
Leishmaniasis	OS or P	15	1	—	2	6
Lentigines	OS	5	1	—	1	—
Lentigo simplex	OS or P	5	1	—	1	—
Lichen planus – hypertrophic	OS	10	1	—	1	—
Lichen sclerosus – vulva	OS	5–10	1	—	2	—
Lichen simplex	OS or P	15–20	1	—	1	—
Lichenoid keratosis – benign	OS	5	1	—	1	—
Lupus erythematosus – discoid	OS	5	1	—	1	—
Lymphangioma	OS	15	1	1–2 mm	2	8
Lymphocytoma cutis	OS	20	1	—	1	—
Melasma	OS	Ice formation	1	—	1	—
Milia	P	5	1	—	1	—
Molluscum contagiosum	P or OS	5	1	—	1	—
Mucocoele – mouth	P	10	1	—	1	—
Myxoid cyst – digital	OS or P	20–30	1	—	1	—
Orf	OS	10	1	—	1	—
Pigmented naevi						
macular	OS	5–10	1	—	1	—
papular	P or OS	15	1	—	2	8
Porokeratosis						
plantaris discreta	OS	Ice formation	1	2 mm	2	2–3
Mibelli	OS	15	1	1 mm	1	—
Prurigo nodularis	OS	10	1	—	1	8
Pruritus ani	OS or P	10	1	—	1	—
Psoriasis – lichenified	OS	10–15	1	—	1	—
Pyogenic granuloma	OS or P	15	1	—	1	—
Rhinophyma	OS	20	1	—	2	8

Table 4.3 continued

Commoner benign lesions Lesion	Technique	Time (secs)	FTC	Margin	Sessions	Interval (weeks)
Rosacea	OS	10	1	—	1	—
Sarcoid – granuloma	OS	10	1	—	1	—
Sebaceous hyperplasia	P or OS	5	1	—	1	—
Seborrhoeic keratosis	OS or P	5–10	1	2 mm	1	—
Skin tags	F or OS	5	1	1 mm	1	—
Solar						
atrophy (fine wrinkles)	OS/Peel	Ice formation	1	—	1	—
keratosis	OS	5	1	—	1	—
lentigo	OS	5	1	—	1	—
Spider naevus	P or OS	10	1	—	1	—
Steatocystoma multiplex	P or OS	10	1	—	2	8
Syringoma	P or OS	5	1	—	2	8
Tattoos	OS	30	1	—	3	8–10
Trichiasis	P	5	1	—	2	4
Trichoepithelioma	P	10–15	1	—	2	8
Venous lakes	P	10	1	—	2	6
Warts						
common	OS	10	1	2–3 mm	3–4	3–4
plane	OS	5	1	1 mm	2	3–4
periungual	OS	15	1	1 mm	3–4	3–4
filiform	OS	5	1	1 mm	1	—
genital	OS	5–10	1	—	3–4	3–4
plantar	OS	20	1	2 mm	3–4	3–4
grouped	OS	30	1	2–3 mm	3–4	4
mosaic	OS	30	1	3–5 mm	4	4
Xanthoma						
xanthelasma	OS	10	1	—	2	8
nodular	OS or P	10	1	2 mm	1	—

P = probe, OS = open spray, F = forceps
These are not fixed treatment times for all lesions but average schedules for average lesions in each diagnostic group.
Treatment times refer to after ice formation.

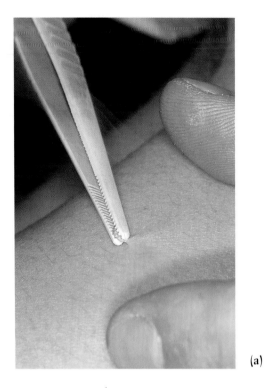
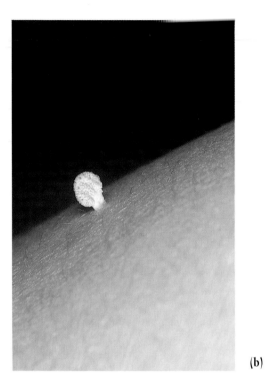

(a)

(b)

Figure 4.23

One effective treatment for skin tags is to dip nontoothed forceps into liquid nitrogen for approximately 30 s and then grasp each tag for about 10 s. **(a)** Frost appearing on forceps and skin tag. **(b)** Frozen tag which will be shed in approximately 10 days.

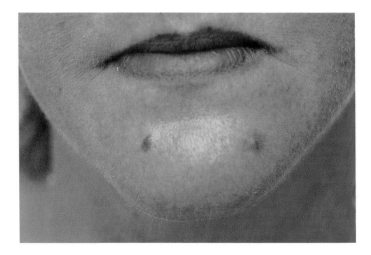

Figure 4.24

Spider angioma and pigmented naevus.

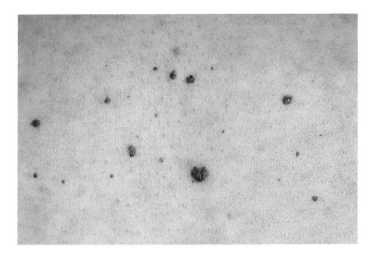

Figure 4.25

Campbell de Morgan spots are common—though treatment is rarely required they respond well to cotton-wool bud or cryoprobe application of approximately 5–10 s depending on lesion size.

not be necessary to destroy the entire lesion and controlled shrinking may be sufficient. For example, when freezing a myxoid cyst the aim is only to fibrose the walls of the sac.

This section lists the common benign tumours that will be encountered by primary care physicians and are suitable for cryosurgical treatment. Some special points concerning diagnosis and treatment are added. It must be stressed that cryosurgery may not be the treatment of choice in each case. Indeed several modes of treatment may exist. But an experienced cryosurgeon may well use liquid nitrogen for all these lesions on occasions.

Suitable lesions

Acne cysts

Superficial cysts will respond to 10–20 seconds of spray (depending on cyst size). Modern antibiotic regimens and oral 13-cis-retinoic acid have reduced the need for this form of treatment.

Acrochordon (skin tag)

Acrochordon is often awkward to treat because of the position—it is difficult to treat lesions uphill. A spray or cotton-wool bud can be directed head on for 5–10 seconds. Another method is to dip forceps into the nitrogen for 20 seconds and then to grasp the stalk of the tag for 10 seconds (Figure 4.23). Tags can also be removed with scissors or destroyed with electrosurgery.

Adenoma sebaceum

Adenoma sebaceum papules are seen in the rare condition of tuberose sclerosis. The facial distribution makes them unsightly. Quite an extensive freeze is needed to remove the larger lesions and the risk of hypopigmentation is great. Laser therapy may therefore be a better choice. Small lesions, however, respond well to nitrogen spray or probe.

Angiomas

Small vascular lesions such as spider naevi (Figure 4.24) and Campbell de Morgan spots

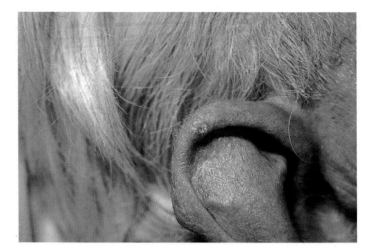

Figure 4.26

Chondrodermatitis helicis is a tender, sometimes very painful nodule on the prominent parts of the pinna.

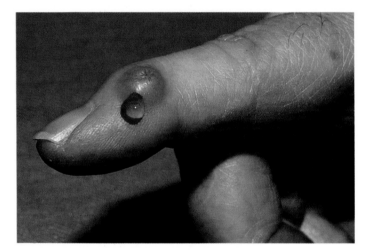

Figure 4.27

Digital myxoid cyst. No method of treatment is uniformly successful. This cyst has been punctured and the gelatinous fluid is being expressed (Epstein technique).

(Figure 4.25) respond to cryosurgery. Accurate localization of the freeze is best accomplished with a cryoprobe and this also allows for some pressure to be applied thus 'emptying' the angioma; no more than 10 seconds total freeze time should be needed, even for the larger lesions.

Chondrodermatitis nodularis helicis

Excision is the most commonly used physical treatment for chondrodermatitis nodularis

helicis but early examples may respond to liquid nitrogen (Figure 4.26).

Condyloma acuminatum (genital warts)

Generally with condyloma acuminatum the patient and any sexual contacts should be screened for other sexually transmitted diseases. The technique is the same as for warts elsewhere but the best results are obtained when topical podophyllin is used in

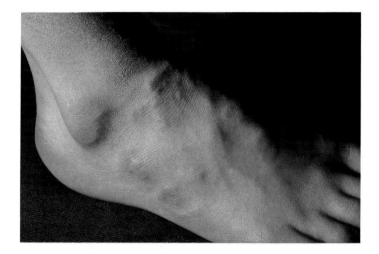

Figure 4.28

The lumpy, ring-shaped appearance of granuloma annulare. Cryosurgery is only successful in approximately 50 per cent of cases—similar treatment regimen as for common warts.

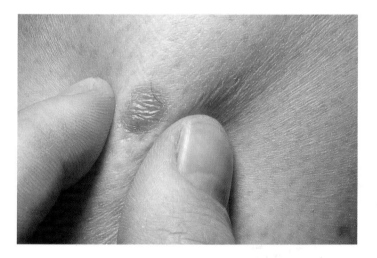

Figure 4.29

Dermatofibroma—these lesions are usually nodular, pink to brown in colour, solitary and asymptomatic; as seen here, the lesion is often attached to deep skin layers and cannot easily be raised up with surrounding skin.

addition. Unfortunately failure and recurrence rates are high.

Digital myxoid cyst

Aggressive cryosurgery is needed to fibrose the walls of digital myxoid cysts (Figure 4.27). After pricking the cyst and expressing the contents a minimum spray of 20 seconds is given; should this prove unsuccessful, up to two 30-second freezes separated by 5 minutes thaw time may be required. This causes considerable morbidity and is best performed by experienced cryosurgeons.

Granuloma annulare

Small lesions may disappear after a 10–20 second freeze—the success rate is no more than 50 per cent (Figure 4.28).

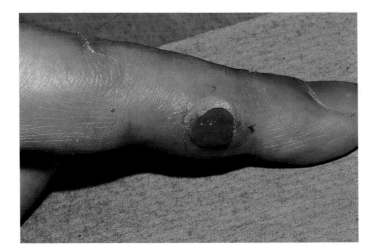

Figure 4.30

Large exuberant pyogenic granuloma. It is wise to obtain histological diagnosis with this type of lesion.

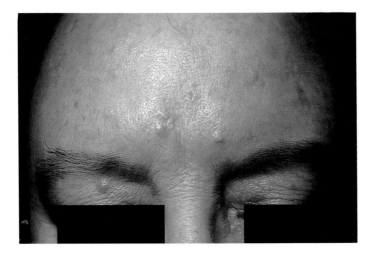

Figure 4.31

Lesions of sebaceous hyperplasia, most commonly on the forehead, can mimic basal cell carcinoma but lack the characteristic 'pearly' colour at its rim.

Histiocytoma (dermatofibroma)

If the diagnosis of histiocytoma (Figure 4.29) is in doubt the nodule should be excised. If not in doubt it can be left untouched, excised or frozen with liquid nitrogen. Cryosurgery may be best for multiple lesions. A prolonged freeze of 30 seconds, using a spray, improves the appearance in approximately 90 per cent of cases.

Ingrowing toenail

When abundant granulation tissue forms with an ingrowing toenail with secondary infection or epithelialization, cryosurgery has a useful place. Using a spray, a single freeze of 30 seconds is carried out.

Keloid

It is wise to attempt small keloids only. Freeze until a 1 mm halo appears on the surrounding skin and repeat this every 3 weeks if necessary. Small 'ear-piercing' keloids respond well but hypopigmentation may follow treatment in dark-skinned individuals.

Labial mucoid cyst

Alternative names for the labial mucoid cyst are mucocoele or mucous retention cyst. This is a common lesion on the lower lip, presenting as a soft red or blue cyst up to 1 cm in diameter. It is particularly suitable for cryoprobe therapy. Lubricant jelly is first applied and the probe is pressed on to the lesion for about 10–20 seconds. No lateral spread of ice is necessary.

Molluscum contagiosum

See above.

Hyperpigmented lesions (benign)

Melanocytes are very sensitive to cold and for this reason it is even more important to be certain of the diagnosis. Inadvertent freezing of a malignant melanoma might well lead, initially, to partial regression and decrease in pigmentation. Whilst apparently improving, however, metastasis could still occur.

There are several forms of increased pigmentation, including simple lentigo and labial macules, which respond well to cryosurgery.

Prurigo nodularis

The intensely itchy nodules of prurigo nodularis are well served by fine nerve endings. Cryosurgery is known to create a degree of anaesthesia and this property has been used in pruritus ani, pruritus vulvae, the itching phases of lichen sclerosus, as well as prurigo nodularis.

Pyogenic granuloma

Cryosurgery can be used to destroy primary pyogenic granuloma (Figure 4.30) but it is wise to obtain tissue for histology if the clinical diagnosis is in any doubt—prominent papular, nodular or pedunculated lesions can

Table 4.3 Some cryosurgery success rates for various benign lesions.

Lesion	Success rate
Viral warts (hand)	75 per cent if treated at 2- or 3-weekly intervals
Verruca	60 per cent cure if treated as for hand warts
Seborrhoeic warts	Despite widespread use little data available. For thin lesions nearly always successful
Dermatofibroma	90 per cent cure or excellent results in study of 35 treated lesions; not the treatment of choice because of pigment charges
Myxoid cysts	86 per cent cure rate
Ingrowing toenail	54 per cent cure rate and up to 64 per cent after second treatment
Tattoos	54 per cent clear after one treatment but morbidity greater than with other modalities of treatment
Chondrodermatitis nodularis helicis	Only 15–20 per cent cure obtained

be broken off while 'iced' and sent for histology. Recurrent lesions however may be suitable for freezing, usually using no more than a single freeze–thaw cycle of 20–30 seconds.

Sebaceous hyperplasia

Sebaceous hyperplasia (Figure 4.31) is most often seen on the central face and can be yellow and shiny, and resemble basal cell carcinoma. The tissue is susceptible to freezing if there is cosmetic concern.

Tattoos

Considerable swelling and morbidity ensues if tattoos are treated. Two cycles of 30 seconds are needed. If the tattoo lies directly over bone it may be very painful afterwards. However, some individuals are desperate to be rid of their stigma. Other methods to consider are excision, infrared coagulation and laser destruction.

Verrucas and other warts

See above.

Xanthelasma

Fatty deposits around the eye are disfiguring. Excision is often possible and some doctors use trichloracetic acid or other corrosive agents touched on to the surface. Liquid nitrogen can be effective but the lax nature of the skin at this site inevitably leads to considerable oedema for 2–3 days after even short freeze times.

Atlas of clinical practice

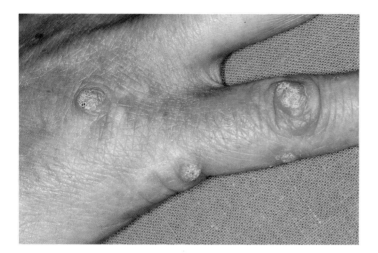

(a)

(b)

Figure 4.32

Clearance of a viral wart 3 weeks after a single 5 s liquid nitrogen spray. (a) The wart prior to treatment. (b) Note some residual erythema but the skin markings now pass through the site, indicating cure.

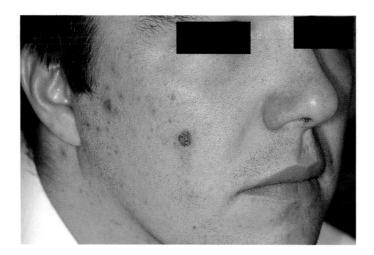

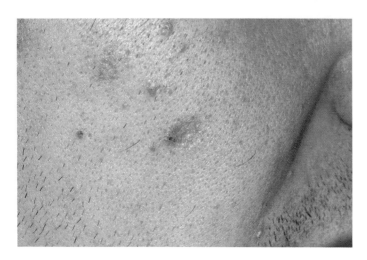

Figure 4.33

(a) Viral wart before cryosurgery.

(b) Three weeks later only slight erythema is visible.

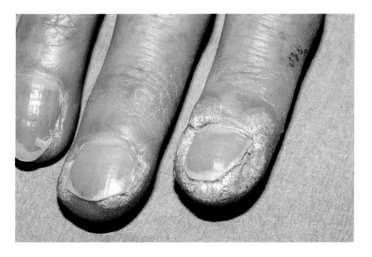

Figure 4.34

(a) Extensive periungual warts.

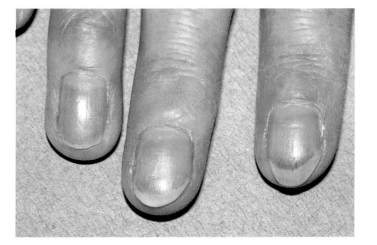

(b) Four months later after four treatments of liquid nitrogen spray. (Courtesy of Dr E C Benton, Edinburgh, UK).

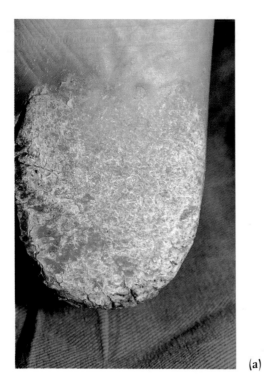

(a)

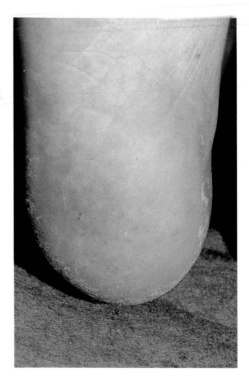

(b)

Figure 4.35

(a) Large mosaic (viral) wart. (b) Four months later following six applications of liquid nitrogen spray.

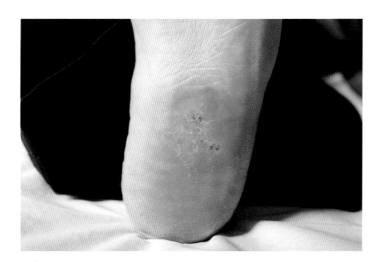

(a)

Figure 4.36
(a) Grouped warts (b) 4 weeks and
(c) 16 weeks after treatment.
(Courtesy of Dr E C Benton,
Edinburgh, UK.)

(b)

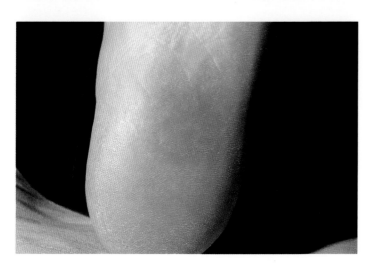

(c)

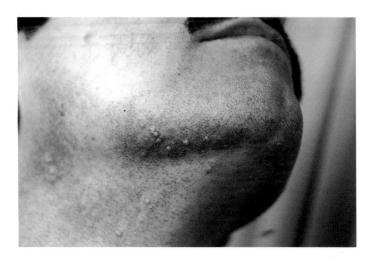

Figure 4.37

(a) Plane warts—beard area.

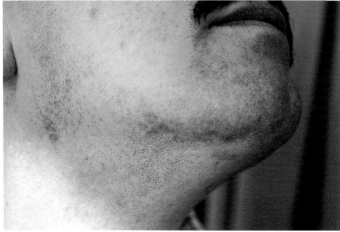

(b) After two applications of liquid nitrogen

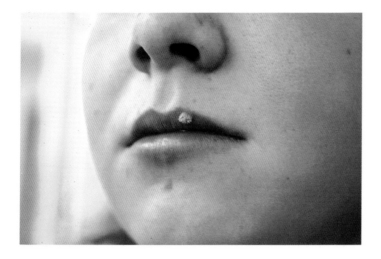

Figure 4.38

(a) Digitate lip wart

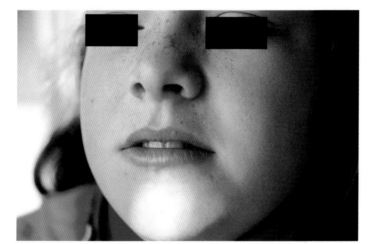

(b) 4 weeks after 10 s liquid nitrogen spray.

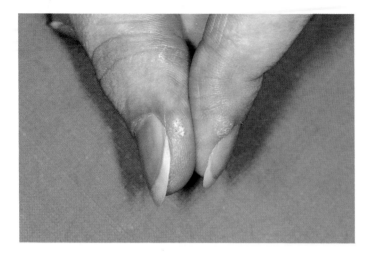

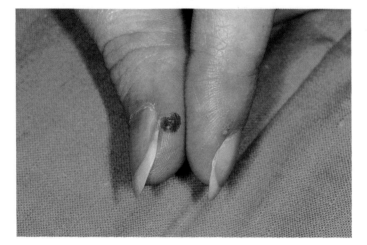

Figure 4.39

(a) Two viral warts prior to treatment.

(b) Only partial response 3 weeks after liquid nitrogen. The inflammatory reaction had, unusually, not settled by this time.

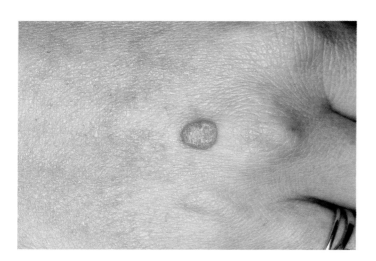

Figure 4.40

(a) Viral wart prior to treatment.

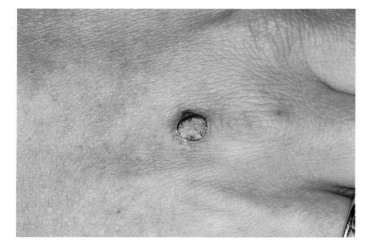

(b) Typical appearance 2 weeks later—some local necrosis has occurred and the deep tissue is about to separate.

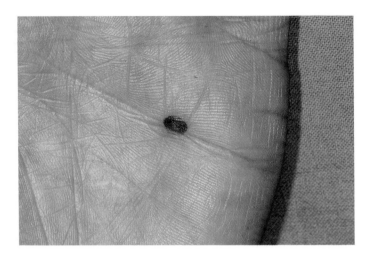

Figure 4.41

(a) Treated wart shortly before the eschar drops off.

(b) One week later the eschar has gone but a nidus of wart is still present (skin creases do not yet traverse the site).

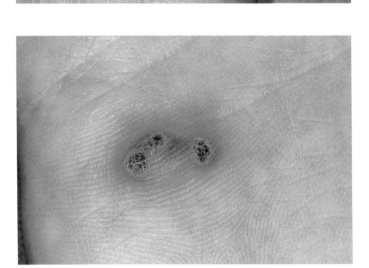

Figure 4.42

Inadequately treated wart—three centres of activity can still be seen after the inflammation has settled.

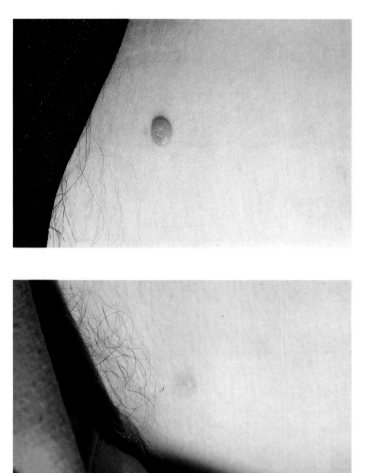

Figure 4.43

(a) Molluscum contagiosum.

(b) Two weeks after 5 s liquid nitrogen spray—only temporary hyperpigmentation remains.

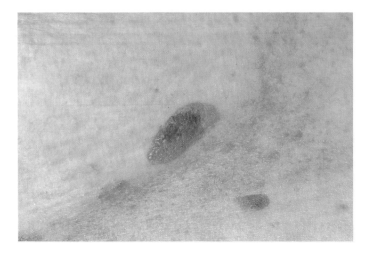

Figure 4.44

(a) Seborrhoeic keratosis—close up view before cyrosurgery.

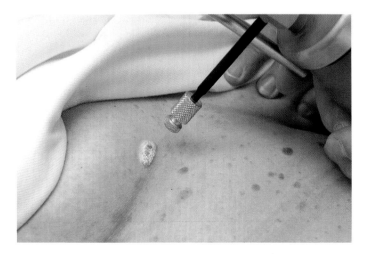

(b) View of area during treatment.

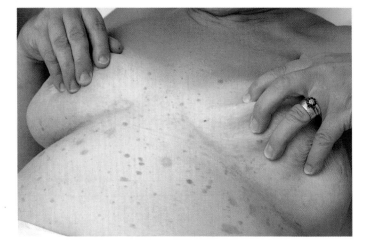

(c) Same site 5 weeks later.

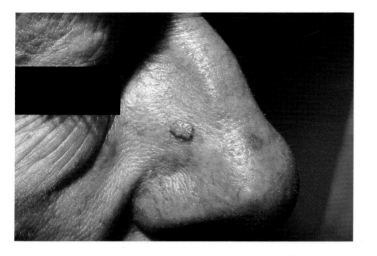

Figure 4.45

(a) Seborrhoeic keratosis of nose.

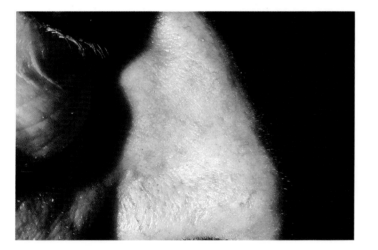

(b) Four weeks after treatment (5 s liquid nitrogen spray).

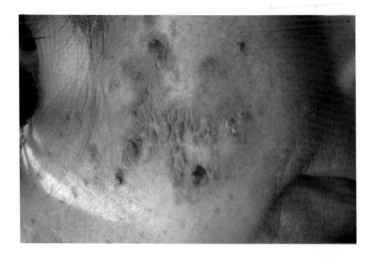

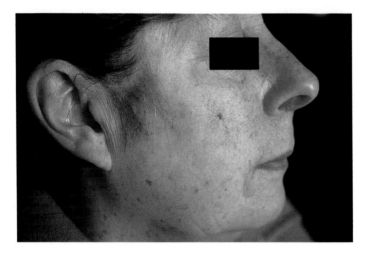

Figure 4.46

(a) Extensive seborrhoeic keratoses of the cheek.

(b) Excellent cosmetic result 6 weeks after liquid nitrogen of 5 s to each area.

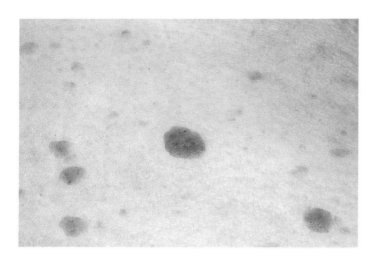

Figure 4.47

(a) Seborrhoeic keratosis.

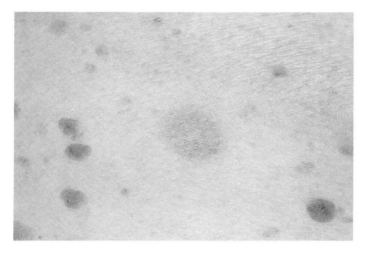

(b) After treatment—temporary post-inflammatory hyperpigmentation.

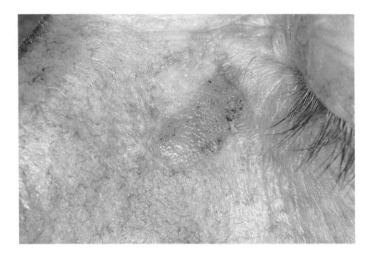

Figure 4.48

(a) Seborrhoeic keratosis—inner canthus.

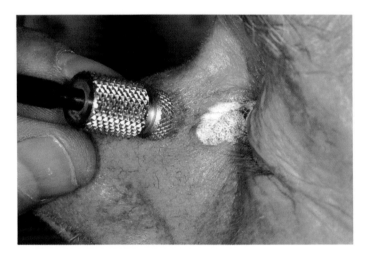

(b) During cryosurgery.

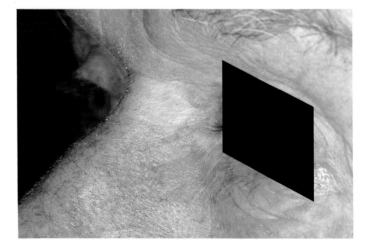

(c) Good result—3 months after therapy.

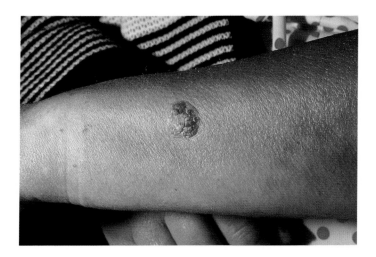

Figure 4.49

(a) Thick, forearm seborrhoeic keratosis.

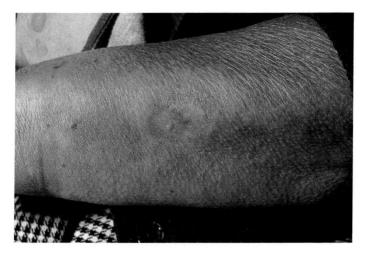

(b) Eight weeks after treatment; slight epidermal atrophy and hypopigmentation—the latter may be permanent.

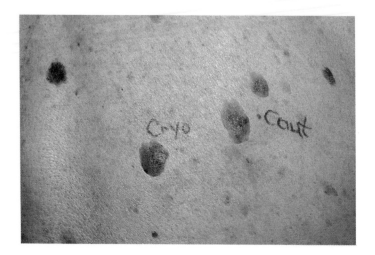

Figure 4.50

(a) Two seborrhoeic keratoses—marked to show the modality of treatment used.

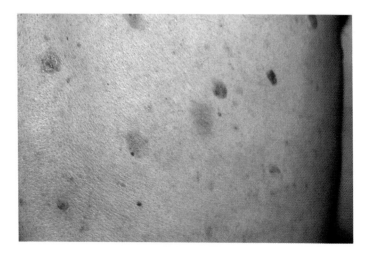

(b) Good results at 6 weeks but more morbidity occurred from cautery.

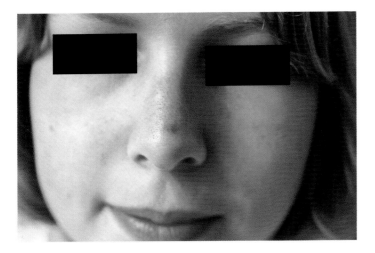

Figure 4.51

(a) Spider angioma (naevus) before liquid nitrogen cryoprobe treatment.

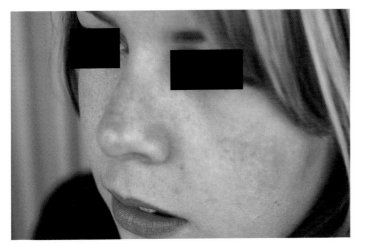

(b) Two months after therapy—only temporary slight reddish hyperpigmentation remains.

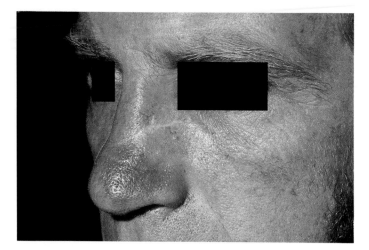

(a)

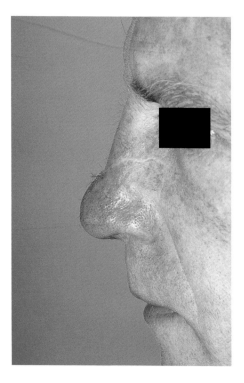

(b)

Figure 4.52

(a) Post-traumatic telangiectasia of the nose—a prominent cosmetic disability. (b) Four months after two treatment sessions—each of 20 s liquid nitrogen spray.

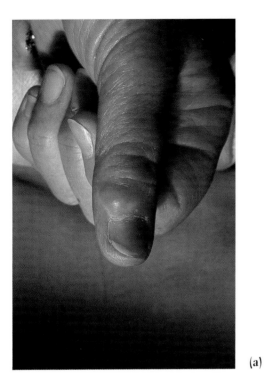 (a)

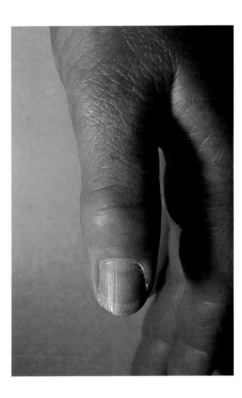 (b)

Figure 4.53

(a) Digital myxoid cyst. (b) Four months after treatment—the lesion was first punctured and the gelatinous contents expressed followed by a single liquid nitrogen spray, inducing ice in the lesion, followed by continuous 20 s spray.

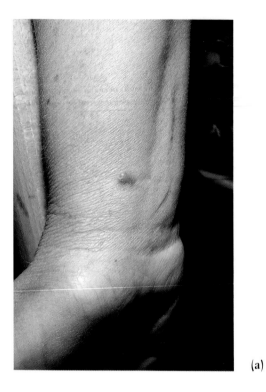 (a)

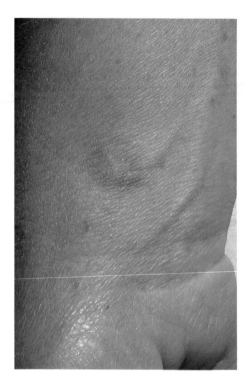 (b)

Figure 4.54

Dermatofibroma (histiocytoma): (a) pretreatment.
(b) Eight weeks after liquid nitrogen spray of 20 s
duration. The lesion was no longer palpable but
the pigmentary change remained visible for over
2 years.

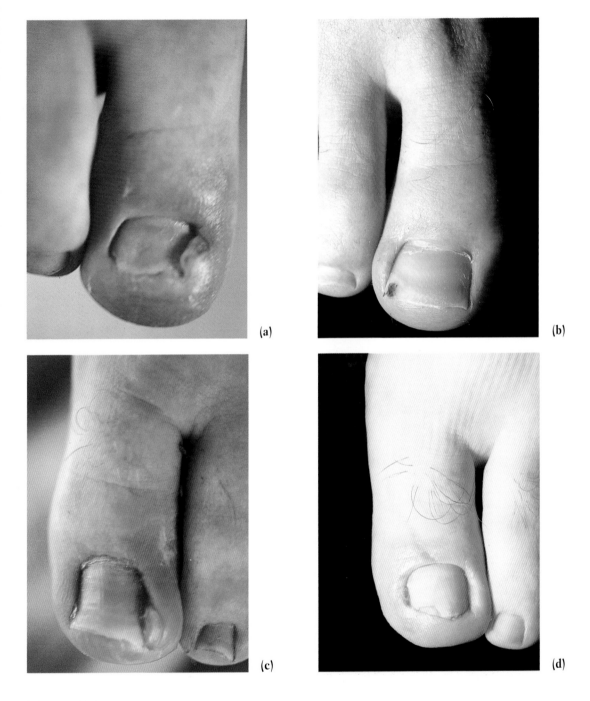

(a)

(b)

(c)

(d)

Figure 4.55

(a) Ingrowing toenail with epithelialized periungual granulation tissue. (b) Eight weeks after a single freeze-thaw cycle (20 s freeze after ice formation) to the abnormal area; (c) Ingrowing nail- (d) 8 weeks after 30 s N_2 spray (spot freeze method)—EMLA cream applied 2 hours before treatment.

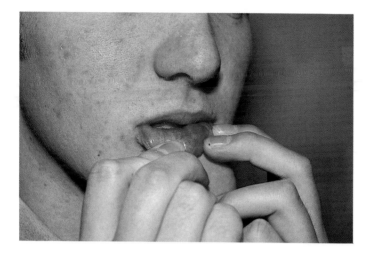

Figure 4.56

(a) Labial mucoid cyst.

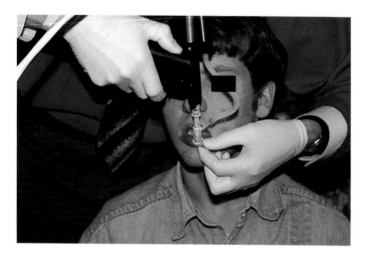

(b) Application of cryoprobe until a halo of ice appeared.

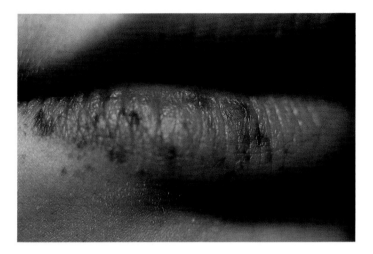

Figure 4.57

(a) Labial lentiginous macules—these may be seen in Laugier–Hunziker syndrome or as an isolated acquired defect.

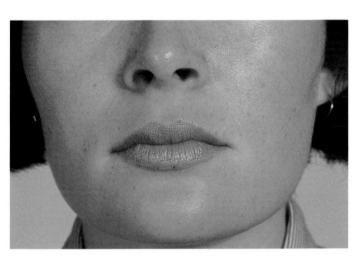

(b) Good result 2 months after liquid nitrogen spray.

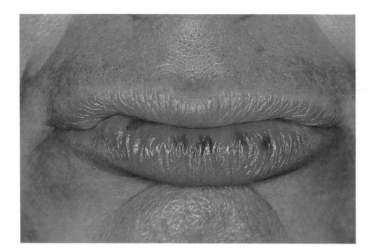

Figure 4.58

(a) Labial lentiginous macules.

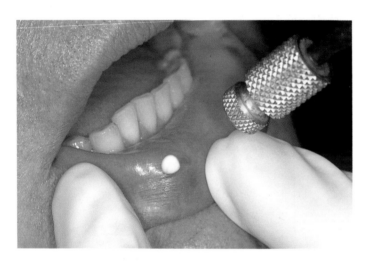

(b) During liquid nitrogen spray.

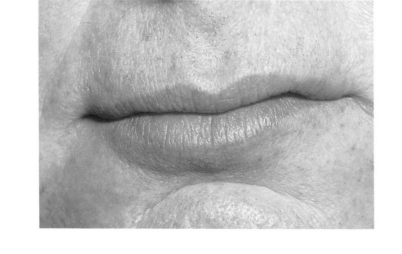

(c) Three months after treatment.

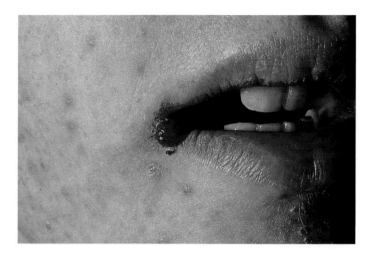

Figure 4.59

Pyogenic granuloma: (a) before treatment.

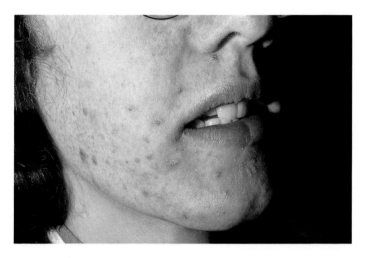

(b) Three weeks after a single 15 s liquid nitrogen spray. If the diagnosis is in doubt the fully 'iced' lesion can be 'broken off' and sent for histology, though this may lead to capillary and venous bleeding for more than 10 minutes.

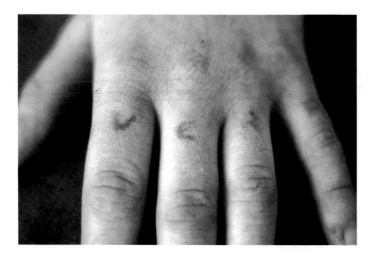

Figure 4.60

(a) Tattoos on fingers of left hand. These can be treated by many surgical methods.

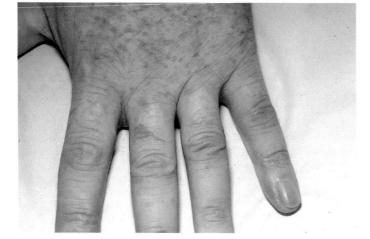

(b) One year after cryosurgery with two freeze-thaw cycles (30 s freeze time). The healing took 6 weeks after initial blistering in all lesions.

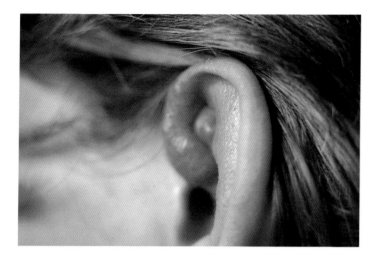

Figure 4.61

(a) Angiolymphoid hyperplasia with eosinophilia.

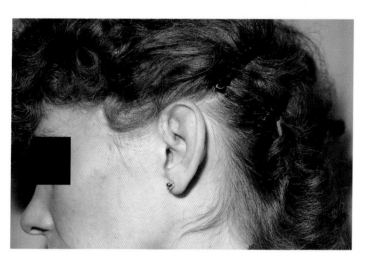

(b) After liquid nitrogen spray.

Bibliography

Bunney MH, Nolan MW, Williams DA (1976), An assessment of methods of treating viral warts by comparative treatment trials based on a standard design, *Br J Dermatol* **94**: 667–679.

Colver GB, Dawber RPR (1984), Tattoo removal using a liquid nitrogen cryospray, *Clin Exp Dermatol* **9**: 364–366.

Dawber RPR, Walker NPJ (1991), Physical and surgical therapy. In: *Textbook of Dermatology*, ed. Champion RH, Burton JL, Ebling J (Oxford, Blackwell) pp 3093–3120.

Kaufman MJ (1993) Full-face cryo-peel termed highly effective in treatment of sun damaged skin, *Cos Derm* **6(9)**: 19–23.

Kuflik EG (1994) Cryosurgery updated. *J Am Acad Dermatol* **31**:925–44.

Sinclair RD, Tzermias C, Dawber RPR (1994) Cosmetic cryosurgery. In: *Cosmetic Dermatology*, eds. Baran R, Maibach H (Martin Dunitz, London) pp 541–550.

5 Premalignant lesions

This chapter deals with those conditions which may possibly progress to malignancy. We include intra epidermal malignancy such as Bowen's and lentigo maligna, both of which may have very long preinvasive gestation phases; indeed, many experienced practitioners have never seen Bowen's disease on skin transform to invasive squamous carcinoma.

- actinic or solar keratosis
- actinic cheilitis
- Bowen's and Bowenoid papulosis
- leucoplakia
- lentigo maligna

Solar keratosis and Bowen's disease are extremely common, have several clinical presentations and are readily amenable to cryosurgery. They both tend to occur as multiple lesions so that treatment may need to be given frequently. Bowen's is most common on the lower legs and needs longer freeze times whereas actinic keratoses tend to be seen on the head and neck and require shorter freeze times.

Leucoplakia may occur on the lips, floor of the mouth and buccal mucosa. There is good agreement that on the floor of the mouth malignant change is likely and may occur as a field change so that extensive surgery is needed. Although the lip may be more amenable to a cryosurgical approach it is considered to be highly specialised and beyond the scope of this book.

Solar keratoses and intraepidermal carcinoma can be confused with other lesions. Both conditions can progress to early neoplastic change with only subtle morphological changes. Whenever there is diagnostic difficulty it is important to take a biopsy before proceeding to cryosurgery. If a malignant tumour is mistakenly treated as premalignant there will be some immediate improvement but the tumour will continue to develop and both patient and physician will be lulled into a false sense of security.

Keratin is a good insulator. The benefits of abrasion or paring the keratin prior to freezing have been examined in Chapter 4. Generally premalignant lesions are less amenable to this approach—the keratin is not always compact and discomfort or bleeding may follow paring. However on occasions, curetting the bulk of a hyperkeratotic lesion before cryosurgery will be helpful and improve the cure rate. A cutaneous horn is a special case because up to 15% will have a malignant base. Here it is necessary to curette or excise and send for histological assessment.

Some practitioners use cryoprobes to treat premalignant lesions. This is a good method for flatter keratoses but if there is an irregular hyperkeratotic surface it will not be possible to obtain good contact. Gels can even this out a little but generally we favour the spray method and the descriptions in the following pages are entirely with this method.

- Lesions on sites with poor skin mobility may be difficult to excise but can be frozen with impunity;
- Lesions on skin which has previously undergone irradiation can be treated by cryosurgery since healing will be satisfactory, in contrast to excision; further radiotherapy would not be appropriate.

Patient information

The side-effects of treating solar keratosis tend to be minimal because they are usually on the head and neck where skin heals well. The after effects of treating Bowen's disease are more severe because longer freezes are needed and the predominant sites on the lower leg heal less well. It is therefore difficult to give general guidelines and the physician must decide at the time which set of instructions to give—those described for benign lesions (see Table 4.1) or those for malignant ones (see Table 6.3).

Patient selection

Initially it is important to choose the right lesions for cryosurgery. The site and other factors will also determine whether it is the most appropriate modality. There are several points in favour of freezing:

- All ages can be treated, even patients in poor health;
- Caucasians respond well as a group because hypopigmentation and hypertrophic scar formation are less of a problem;
- Even in sites where keloids are common (e.g. anterior chest and upper arm) it is safe to use cryosurgery;
- Those on anticoagulants and those allergic to local anaesthetic can be treated safely;

Solar keratosis (SK)

These are areas of adherent hyperkeratosis developing in sun-exposed skin, usually occurring at or after middle age. Fair-skinned people are more often affected. This is more obvious and seen at an earlier age in those who live in areas of high sun exposure. The problem has become enormous in Australia, New Zealand and the southern United States but young people everywhere have been receiving higher doses of ultraviolet radiation on foreign holidays for many years and in this group the incidence is also rising.

Keratoses may also follow ionizing radiation, radiant heat, exposure to tar and ingestion of inorganic arsenic.

These keratoses probably have malignant potential, though the risk is small. Even if the keratoses arc not premalignant, they are certainly associated with a risk of basal and squamous cell carcinoma. The huge majority of lesions never become malignant; on the other hand, the majority of squamous carcinomas arising on sun-exposed skin are probably preceded by a dysplastic keratosis. Careful study of solar keratoses in an Australian population revealed that many of them simply disappear.

Clinical problems of SK

The patient may seek advice for several reasons:

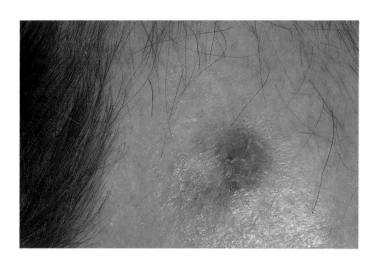

Figure 5.1

Early solar keratosis—only slight scale present.

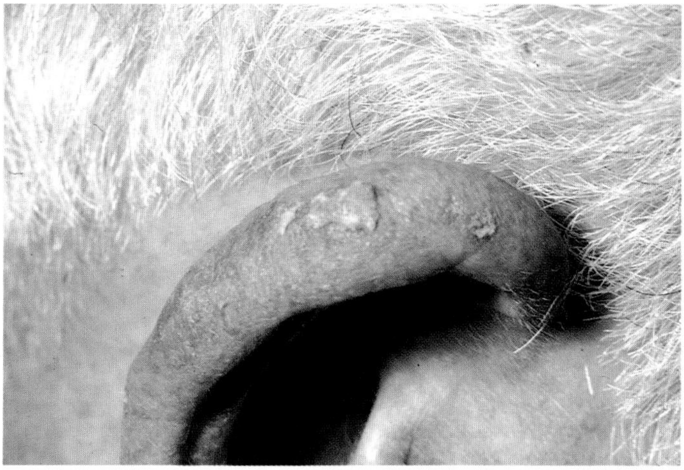

Figure 5.2

Solar keratosis with more prominent keratosis (compare Figure 5.1).

- Cancer worries
- Cosmetic worries
- Soreness or itching
- Bleeding from minor trauma
- Rapid growth with malignant change.

They may have this appearance for many months with little or no scale (Figure 5.1). Usually, however, adherent scale becomes a feature. The sites more often affected are the backs of the hands, forearms and upper face. The main varieties are described below.

Clinical varieties of SK

Solar keratoses often begin as almost indiscernible telangiectatic areas with scaling.

Common

A yellow or brown rough scale is the main feature (Figure 5.2). They are frequently

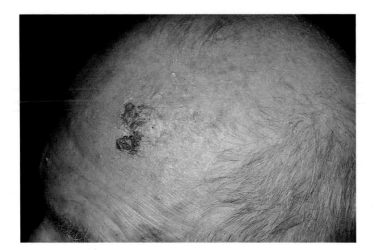

Figure 5.3

Solar keratosis—a large hyperkeratotic lesion with many smaller lesions on the scalp.

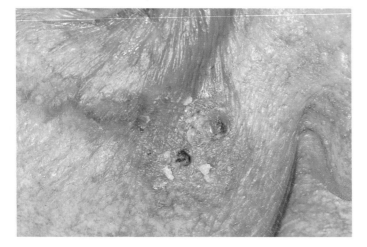

Figure 5.4

Solar keratosis—some areas have shed the hyperkeratosis.

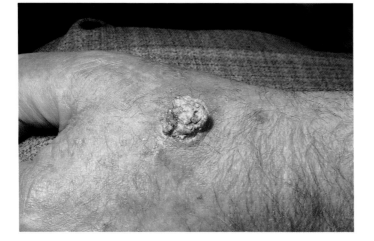

Figure 5.5

Cutaneous horn type of solar keratosis.

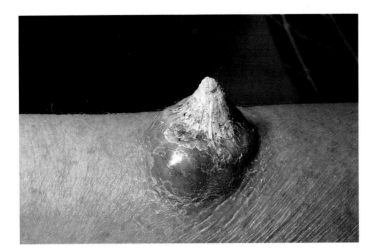

Figure 5.6

Keratoacanthoma—regular raised margin with central 'crater' filled with horny keratin. A self-healing type of epithelioma that usually remits spontaneously. It responds poorly to cryosurgery and is better curetted or excised to obtain histological diagnosis.

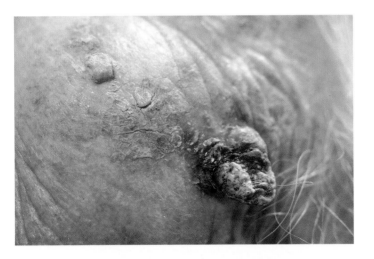

Figure 5.7

Cutaneous horny lesion with an indurated base—histologically an early squamous carcinoma.

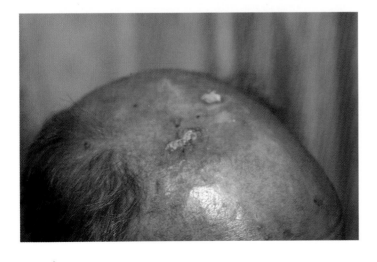

Figure 5.8

The upper lesion is a solar keratosis but the lower lesion was a histologically proven early squamous carcinoma.

multiple with the overall effect often described as like touching sandpaper (Figure 5.3). The surrounding skin may be red (Figure 5.4), atrophic and wrinkled.

Pigmented

This type may be almost flat or raised and the pigment raises doubts regarding a melanocytic lesion. However, the typical scaly roughness is almost always present on pigmented solar keratoses—if doubt exists then biopsy or excision is required.

Cutaneous horn and early carcinoma

Several pathologies, as well as solar keratosis (Figure 5.5), may underlie this structure, e.g. viral wart, seborrhoeic keratosis and keratoacanthoma (Figure 5.6). Up to 15% may be early squamous carcinoma (Figure 5.7).

Features which may indicate malignant change are an indurated base and rapid growth (Figure 5.8). Biopsy does not always confirm malignancy but it is a wise precaution to biopsy or excise lesions if these features are seen.

Treatment of solar keratosis

Cryosurgery is not always the best method but remains a quick and effective one. Sometimes a combination of freezing and topical preparations will contain a difficult situation as is seen in fair skinned individuals with a lifetime of excessive ultraviolet exposure. Such people may have fifty or more new keratoses a year.

- Multiple small areas can be managed with 5–10% salicyclic acid in white soft paraffin.
- Topical 5-fluorouracil is good for extensive changes. The package insert is fairly

dear but some specialists prefer to use it on a one week in four basis to all 'exposed' head and hand sites as prophylaxis. Whichever protocol is followed it is important to wash the cream off after 12 hours and to avoid contact with the eyes.

- Topical tretinoin preparations are used around the world, as prophylaxis and treatment for multiple small lesions but are rather irritant.
- Curettage and cautery (or electrodessication) is a well-tried and successful therapy, particularly for large lesions.
- Cryosurgery. Cotton-wool buds or sprays are suitable here. The spot-freeze method is effective and reproducible. So much variation is found between barely palpable lesions and large indurated keratoses that it is impossible to give firm guidelines. Having established an icefield the freeze should be maintained for at least 5 seconds. This may have to be extended to 15 seconds for bulkier lesions. Some authors recommend the paint brush pattern of spraying (10–30 seconds) and report excellent results.
- The eye should be protected if spraying is carried out to periocular lesions.

Since these are possibly premalignant (clinically 'benign') lesions it is permissible to be conservative when delineating the margins. Only a 1 mm rim of apparently healthy tissue need be included in the icefield; it is best to mark this out in ink before commencing treatment. Recurrences can be managed by further freezing at a later date. If, on the other hand, a keratosis regrows quickly it may be more appropriate to curette or excise at the next visit in order to check the histology.

Actinic cheilitis

Intense and prolonged exposure to ultraviolet light may lead to changes on the lower lip.

It begins with dryness and then thickened grey-white plaques. Variable inflammation and crusting follow. It should be differentiated from lichen planus, lupus erythematosus and leucoplakia. Many publications on cryotherapy place actinic cheilitis and leucoplakia together. They both have malignant potential but are best kept separate. Small areas of actinic cheilitis can be treated by cryosurgery using the same sort of treatment schedules as for Bowen's disease. However more extensive changes may be resistant and one may have to resort to surgical lip shaving with mucosal advancement or carbon dioxide laser ablation.

Bowen's disease (carcinoma in situ)

This begins as an area of pink, scaly or crusted skin that has a slow radial growth pattern. The cellular changes are neoplastic but are localized entirely within the epidermis. When the changes breach the basement membrane the lesion is considered to have undergone malignant transformation into a squamous carcinoma. This develops in 3–5 per cent of untreated patients. The aetiology of Bowen's disease is not clear but most lesions are on sun-exposed skin; there is also a known association with previous arsenic ingestion. However, any part of the body can be affected. In practice, many patches of Bowen's disease are seen on the leg below the knee in women with fair skin. The first change is a small red scaly area, which gradually enlarges. The margin is clear but often irregular and the surface has a white or yellowy scale. Several lesions may appear either together or widely scattered. The morphological changes of an individual lesion may be similar to those of a small psoriatic plaque.

Clinical problems

The patient may seek advice for several reasons:

- Cancer worries;
- Horny keratin catching on tights or other clothing;
- Erosion, oozing, rapid growth (and so on), indicating possible malignant transformation.

Clinical varieties

Common type

An early pink scaly plaque (Figures 5.9–5.11) may look similar to a patch of psoriasis. The edge is often scalloped. Some lesions become very large (Figure 5.12).

Hyperkeratotic

The surface may be heaped up into a horn or a thick plaque. Scale may be lost in the centre (Figure 5.13).

Erythroplasia of Queyrat

This is on the glans penis and has a red velvety surface appearance. It should be differentiated from Zoons (plasma cell) balanitis and a biopsy is needed before cryosurgery to exclude progression to invasive malignancy.

Treatment

Several methods give satisfactory cure rates. The most suitable will depend on the size and site of the plaque and the general condition of

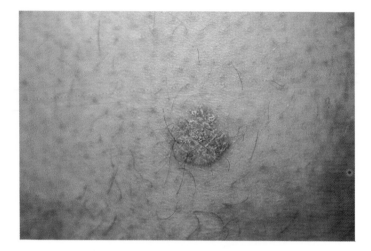

Figure 5.9

Bowen's disease—a pink, scaly 'psoriasiform' patch.

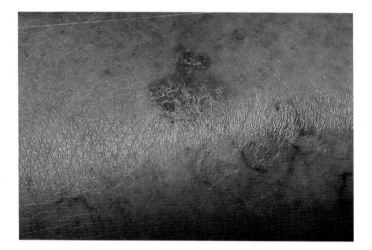

Figure 5.10

Bowen's disease of the shin.

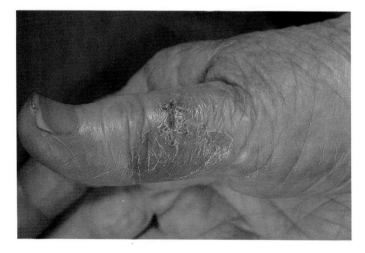

Figure 5.11

Bowen's disease of the thumb.

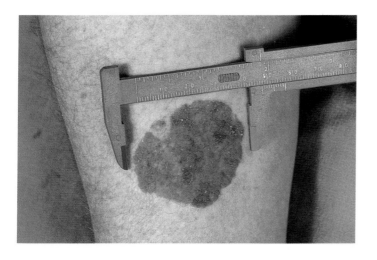

Figure 5.12

Bowen's disease—a large lesion.

the patient. In elderly individuals it may be most appropriate to simply make the diagnosis and explain the need for watchfulness. Symptomatic lesions would, of course, warrant treatment.

- Excision is appropriate if the lesion is small, enabling complete histological assessment.
- Electrosurgery, usually associated with preceding curettage.
- Topical 5-fluorouracil, usually as a 5 per cent cream.
- Cryosurgery. Sprays are better than cotton-wool buds here. After an icefield is established it is best to maintain it for 20–30 seconds. Only a single freeze–thaw cycle is needed. A rim of 2 mm of healthy

tissue should be included. For small early lesions this is a simple matter. Larger examples should be divided up into overlapping circles. Each circle can then be treated with a 20 second freeze–thaw cycle (Figure 5.14). One area can be frozen and left to heal for a few weeks before dealing with the remainder if there is a possibility of delayed healing. When correctly used cryosurgery can probably now be designated as the treatment of choice for most cases of skin Bowen's disease. Markedly hyperkeratotic lesions can be excised or debulked by curettage prior to cryosurgery.

Intraepidermal carcinoma often extends down the appendageal epithelium of hair follicles and will be protected from superficial freezing or electrosurgery. Recurrence is then quite common, with new areas appearing even in the middle of previously treated sites. Further liquid nitrogen can be carried out; excision may be preferable.

Bowen's disease is often seen on the lower leg in older age groups, with a female preponderance. Aggressive cryosurgery can easily lead to ulcers, with delayed healing. There is only a small risk of malignant transformation so careful judgement must be exercised when deciding who and how to treat.

Erythroplasia of Queyrat (Bowen's disease of the glans penis or vulval epithelium) is an uncommon disease. There are no big studies which compare cure rates for different treatments or which look at optimal freezing times with cryosurgery. However, most authors are encouraging about the effectiveness of liquid nitrogen in this disease. The absence of hairs on mucosal skin means that the abnormal cells do not delve below the basement membrane. A 30 second freeze thaw cycle is recommended and there are no concerns about healing which is rapid, leaving a functionally and cosmetically excellent result. Vulval dysplasia of human papilloma virus type is relatively resistant to cryosurgery.

Bowenoid papulosis occurs on the genital epithelium and also the surrounding skin. Lesions are usually multiple, smaller than 1 cm and red to brown in colour. There appears to be an associated HPV infection and there is a small risk of squamous carcinoma of the genital tract. Generally in young immunocompetent individuals there is little risk and spontaneous recovery may be seen; in others, especially older patients it proves a more difficult problem. Cryosurgery is effective in many cases using the same treatment protocols as for Bowen's disease elsewhere.

Table 5.1 **Practical treatment schedules.**

Premalignant lesions *Lesion*	*Technique*	*Time (secs)*	*FTC*	*Margin*	*Sessions*	*Interval (weeks)*	*Response*
Actinic cheilitis	OS	20	1	—	1	—	95–96%
Bowen's disease							
Skin	OS	15–30	1	2 mm	2	12	85–99%
Penile (erythroplasia)	OS	20	1	2 mm	1	—	97%
Bowenoid papulosis	OS	10	1	2 mm	4	6	94–97%
Keratoacanthoma	OS	30	2	5 mm	2	6	50–60%
Lentigo maligna	OS	30	1	3 mm	1	—	84–94%
Leucoplakia	OS	20	1	2–3 mm	1–2	8	>90%

OS = open spray.
These are guidelines for 'average' lesions only. They are not necessarily 'treatments of choice'.

Lentigo maligna

Though preinvasive (melanoma in situ) Lentigo maligna is described in conjunction with the invasive form, lentigo maligna melanoma in Chapter 6. In the view of many practitioners it should be managed as more akin to malignancy than carcinoma-in-situ— in view of the perceived difficulty of defining the pure preinvasive form. The work of Yell et al (1996) suggests that the clinician's diagnostic acumen in excluding invasion on visual and palpation criteria is adequate for routine practice.

How effective is cryosurgery?

With a premalignant disease, high cure rates must be weighed against side-effects. No one will thank the physician who guarantees a cure at the expense of a slow-healing, painful ulcer. It is therefore justifiable to introduce a modicum of conservatism into this treatment.

The majority of dermatologists in the western world treat solar keratoses and Bowen's disease with liquid nitrogen cryosurgery but very few have reported failure or recurrence rates. One series of over 1000 treated solar keratoses reported a 98 per cent cure rate; in a study of cryosurgery in the treatment of 128 cases of Bowen's disease only 0.8 per cent recurred. Other people have less good results but do not publish them. In some patients Bowen's disease appears to be a field change and new areas of disease arise beyond the edge of the treated area. In these cases, it is by no means certain that any other modality would be more successful.

Atlas of clinical practice

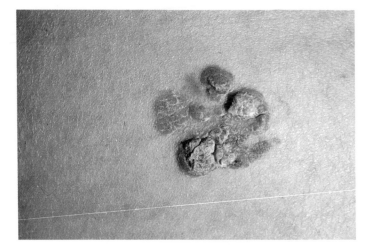

Figure 5.13

Bowen's disease—an irregularly hyperkeratotic patch: (a) before cryosurgery.

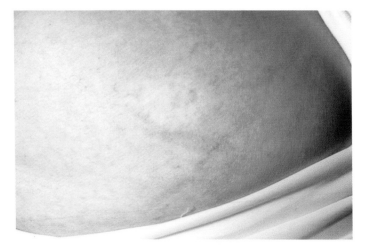

(b) After cryosurgery—treated by one freeze (20 s)–thaw cycle.

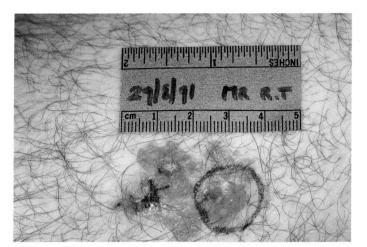

Figure 5.14

Bowen's disease: (a) before cryosurgery.

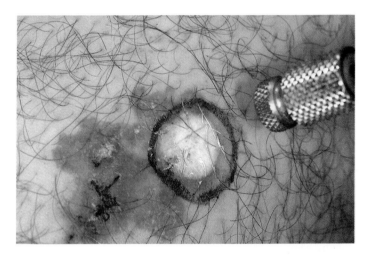

(b) During cryosurgery.

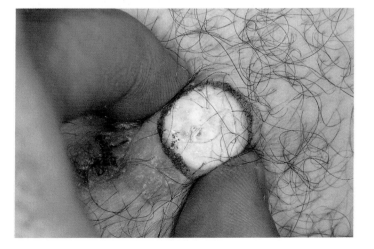

(c) During cryosurgery. The icefield is palpated to ensure full skin thickness is uniformly frozen.

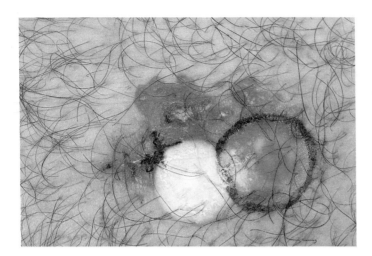

Figure 5.14 *(continued)*

(d) During cryosurgery.

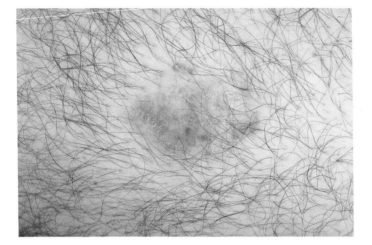

(e) After treatment by cryosurgery—using overlapping fields of freezing—see Chapter 3.

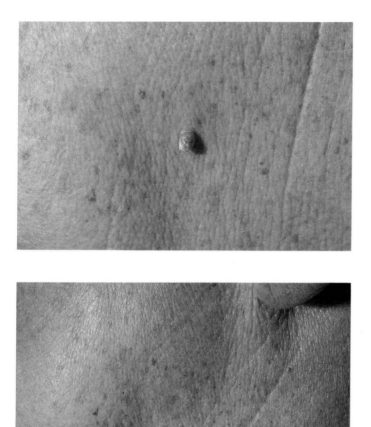

Figure 5.15

(a) A cutaneous horn on exposed skin.

(b) After 5 s liquid nitrogen spray.

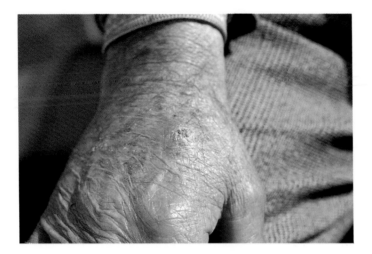

Figure 5.16

(a) Solar keratosis on the dorsum of the hand.

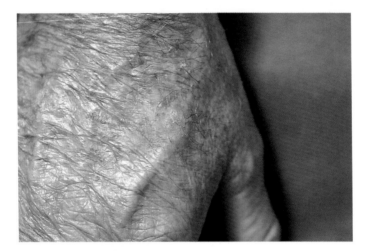

(b) After treatment—5 s liquid nitrogen spray.

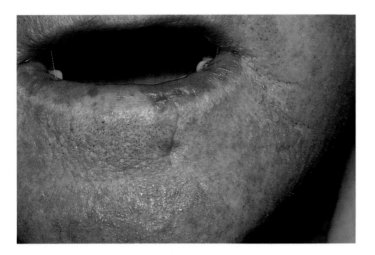

Figure 5.17

(a) Solar keratosis (atrophic) associated with diffuse actinic cheilitis.

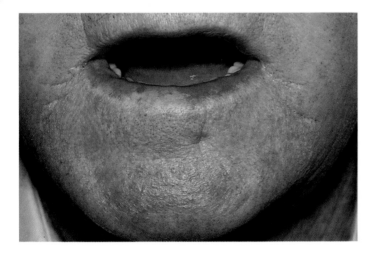

(b) After cryosurgery—good response; the remaining red erosive area can easily be retreated. (NB any indurated areas must be biopsied to exclude squamous carcinoma—not present in this case.)

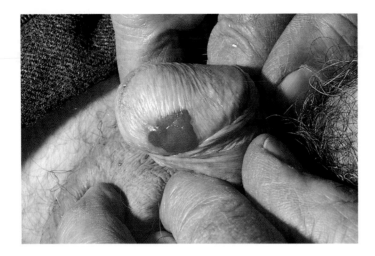

Figure 5.18

(a) Bowen's disease of the glans penis (erythroplasia of Queyrat).

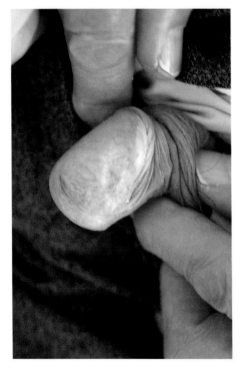

(b) After treatment—one freeze (30 s)–thaw cycle. No recurrence was seen up to 6 years later.

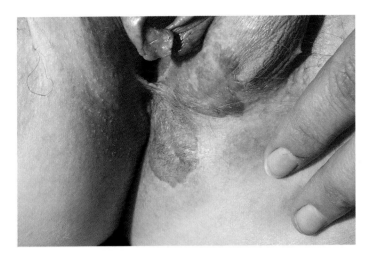

Figure 5.19

(a) Pigmented Bowen's disease of the vulva and perineum.

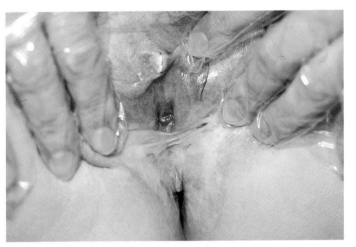

(b) After cryosurgery—a single freeze (30 s)–thaw cycle was used. The normal stretching of skin shows that no inelastic scar tissue has occurred, though hypopigmentation is obvious.

Bibliography

Dawber RPR, Walker NPJ (1991), Physical and surgical therapy. In: *Textbook of dermatology*, ed. Champion RH, Burton JL, Ebling J (Oxford, Blackwell) pp 3093–3120.

Graham GF, Clark LC (1985), Statistical update in cryosurgery for cancers of the skin. In: *Cryosurgery for skin cancer and cutaneous disorders*, ed. Zacarian SA (St Louis, Mosby Co) pp 298–305.

Holt PJ (1988), Cryotherapy for skin cancer: results over a 5-year period using liquid nitrogen spray cryosurgery, *Br J Dermatol*, **119**:231–240.

Kuflik EG (1994), Cryosurgery updated. *J Am Acad Dermatol* **31**:925–44.

Lubritz RR, Smolewski SA (1982), Cryosurgery cure rate of actinic keratoses, *J Am Acad Dermatol*, **7**:631–632.

Yell JA, Baigrie C, Dawber RPR, Millard PR, Goodacre TE (1996), Cryotherapy for lentigo maligna—is clinical acumen combined with a single punch biopsy good enough for staging. *J Eur Acad Dermatol Venereol* **7(1)**: 39–44.

6 Malignant lesions

With appropriate selection of patients and tumours, adequate equipment and proper techniques, cryosurgery is an excellent therapeutic modality for the treatment of skin malignancy. Indeed it is the treatment of choice for some skin cancers and a good alternative in other settings. As with other established techniques such as conventional surgery, electrosurgery, radiotherapy and histographic surgery (Mohs' technique), it has its own special advantages and limitations.

tumour-free margin around the lesion, in order to ensure adequate destruction peripherally. To achieve adequate depth of cryonecrosis for most tumours one should carry out a double 30 second freeze–thaw cycle (spot freeze method), with a minimum 5 minute thaw period between each freeze. Basal cell carcinomas away from the head and neck respond equally well to a single freeze-thaw cycle (Mallon and Dawber, 1996). The scientific basis and technique involved have already been discussed (Chapters 2 and 3).

Principles of treatment

The aim when treating skin cancers with cryosurgery is destruction of the lesion at the first treatment. In order to accomplish this, the tumour must be frozen to sufficient depth and with adequate peripheral margins so that no focus of malignancy remains untreated.

Most failures in cryosurgical treatment of skin cancers are due to poor technique rather than the nature of the lesion. Liquid nitrogen, with its boiling point of –196°C, is the most reliable refrigerant for consistent cell destruction. When preparing the field for treatment, one should include a minimum 3 mm

Patient selection

The decision as to whether to treat a malignant lesion by cryosurgery depends on several factors. These include the size of the lesion, its site and the histopathology. In addition, the patient's age and state of health are important. The ease with which a patient can attend for a particular treatment may also be relevant—for example, one can treat elderly housebound patients by cryosurgery in their own homes. Table 6.1 summarizes the histological types of skin cancer, the morphological features and the selection of patients for whom cryosurgery is most suitable.

Table 6.1   Tumours and patients most suitable for cryosurgery.

Types of skin cancer

Superficial basal cell carcinoma
Nodular or ulcerated basal cell carcinoma
Basal cell naevus syndrome
Small, well-differentiated squamous cell
    carcinoma arising in actinic keratoses

Selection of tumours

Tumours under 2 cm in diameter, with the
    exception of multicentric superficial basal cell
    carcinomas which are usually wide-spreading
Tumours with definable margins
Tumours overlying cartilage and bone
Tumours invading the ear, eyelid and nose
    (avoiding chondronecrosis, lacrimal obstruction
    and mutilating surgical excision)
Infected tumours
Recurrent tumours from previous radiotherapy

Selection of patients

Patients of all ages, but especially those of poor
    risk for surgery and for general anaesthesia
Patients with a history of infectious jaundice or
    other serologically transmitted diseases

Table 6.2   Tumours less suitable for cryosurgery.

Tumours over 2 cm in diameter
Recurrent tumours (with the exception of post
    radiotherapy)
Tumours with a high recurrence rate, e.g.
    tumours situated on the nasolabial fold and
    periauricular areas
Tumours of the feet and lower legs where the
    time of healing can be protracted
Tumours with the histopathological diagnosis of
    morphoeic or sclerotic, metatypical or
    mixed type

Table 6.3   Advice sheet following cryosurgery for malignant lesions.

PATIENT INFORMATION LEAFLET

CRYOSURGERY

After cryosurgery the treated area will swell and
    weep considerably, but this can be reduced by
    the application of clobetasol propionate 0.5 per
    cent cream and a gauze dressing which should
    be held in place by adhesive tape; the cream
    can be reapplied daily for 4–5 days to minimize
    the early redness, swelling and soreness.
The wound should form a hard, dry, black adher-
    ent crust after 10–14 days. It may be anything
    from a week to a month or more before it sepa-
    rates to leave a pink scar that ultimately
    becomes white.
There should be relatively little pain after the
    procedure, but aspirin 300–600 mg, 4–6 hourly
    can be taken if required. In the case of aspirin
    intolerance, paracetamol (acetaminophen) may
    be used instead. Severe pain or swelling may
    indicate the presence of secondary infection,
    when a course of antibiotics may be prescribed
    by your doctor.
If any problems arise in connection with your
    cryosurgery, please contact your doctor
    (Telephone no:...... extension......).

Table 6.2 summarizes the features that make
a tumour less suitable for cryosurgery

Patient information

In contrast to benign lesions, which only
require a short, single freeze and no anaesthetic, cystic or solid types of basal cell carcinoma often require local anaesthetic and a
double 30 second freeze–thaw cycle. The end
result is usually excellent, but the reaction of
the malignant and surrounding tissues is
considerable and complete healing takes
several weeks.

Before treatment it is, therefore, most important to give a thorough explanation to the patient of all the possible side-effects. This should cover the initial swelling, degree of pain and the subsequent care of the treated area. The advice is best reinforced by an information sheet, which the patient and relatives can read at their leisure. Table 6.3 is an example of such a leaflet.

Tumour histopathology

Whilst it is safe to undertreat a benign skin lesion, the degree of freeze given to a malignant lesion is crucial. Whenever the diagnosis is in doubt, a pretreatment biopsy should be performed. The biopsy, under local anaesthetic, may be conducted as an incisional edge biopsy, a punch biopsy or by curettage. Taking the biopsy before undertaking cryosurgery has two important advantages:

- It may determine the cryosurgical technique required, e.g. a deeply infiltrating basal cell carcinoma or the more invasive squamous cell carcinoma need a double 30 second freeze–thaw cycle whereas a superficial basal cell carcinoma may require no more than a single 20 second freeze–thaw cycle. The patient can be informed accordingly.
- Healing of normal surrounding tissue and removal of any biopsy suture is achieved before cryosurgery is undertaken. The possibility of bleeding during cryosurgery is reduced. Bleeding not infrequently occurs during the thaw period if a biopsy is carried out immediately prior to cryofreeze or as a freeze biopsy.

The preceding paragraphs have highlighted the basic rules for the cryosurgical treatment of malignant skin lesions; in practice some minor variations and modifications in the techniques used for different skin malignancies will be required. If one is at all unsure of the length of freeze to give a particular lesion, good general rules are:

- Undertreat benign lesions
- Overtreat malignant lesions.

Basal cell carcinoma

Varieties of basal cell carcinoma (BCC)

There are three main types:

- Nodular
- Superficial
- Morphoeic.

Nodular lesions are raised with translucent pearly borders. Small telangiectatic vessels may course across the surface. They may be ulcerated centrally, giving rise to the typical 'rodent ulcer' (Figure 6.1).

Superficial BCCs start as flat, red, slightly scaly patches, which spread and become more scaly. They may have a 'whipcord' edge. They generally occur on the trunk (Figure 6.2).

Morphoeic BCCs appear as waxy, indurated plaques. The borders are indistinct (Figure 6.3).

Although these descriptions fit most BCCs, it is not uncommon to find a small papule, cyst or crust that histologically reveals a basal cell carcinoma. It is therefore important to biopsy any persistent acquired lesion in the older patient.

Superficial spreading basal cell carcinomas of the type often seen on the trunk of elderly patients (Figure 6.4) (i.e. sun exposure is not a factor), lesions of the basal cell naevus syndrome and small lesions on X-ray damaged skin (Figure 6.5) may be treated with a single freeze–thaw cycle. Swelling and morbidity will be less than after the double

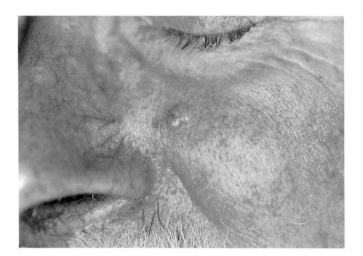

Figure 6.1
Typical 'rodent ulcer' of the face.

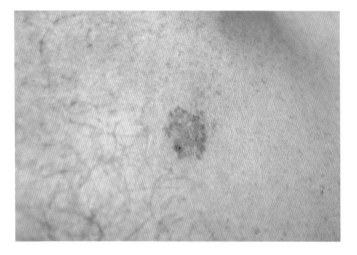

Figure 6.2
Superficial BCC of the chest.

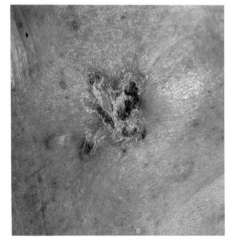

Figure 6.3
Morphoeic BCC of cheek—note indistinct borders.

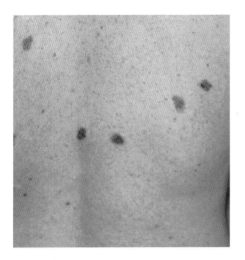

Figure 6.4
Multiple superficial BCC's on trunk.

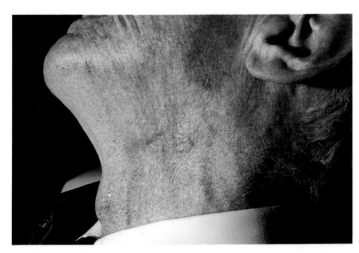

Figure 6.5
(a) Superficial BCC of X-ray damaged skin.

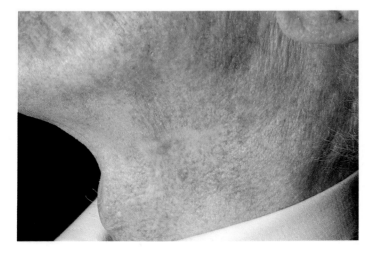

(b) Readily treated by cryosurgery—12 weeks after a single freeze (30 s)–thaw cycle.

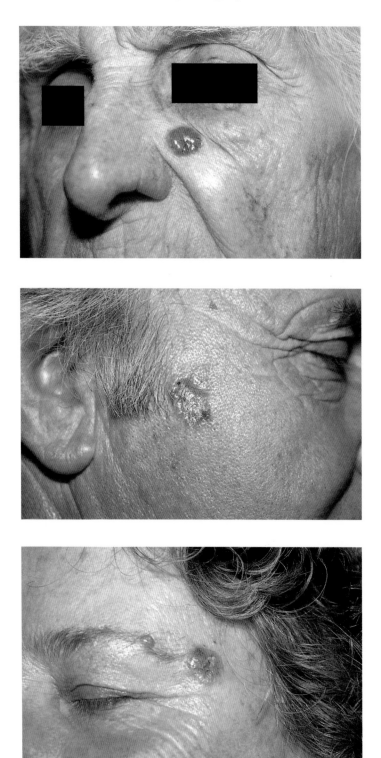

Figure 6.6 (a–i)

Various types of BCC.

(a)

(b)

(c)

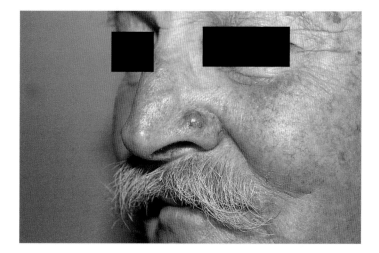

(d)

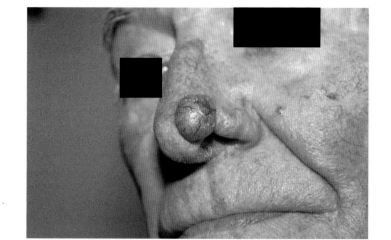

(e)

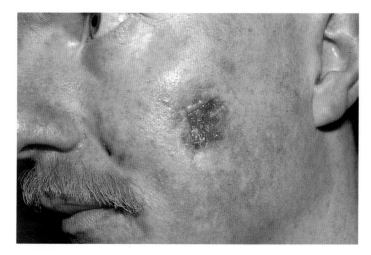

(f)

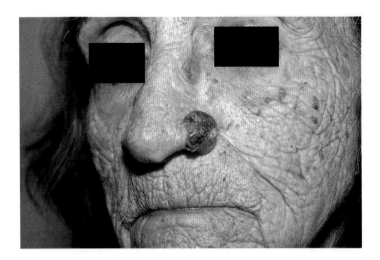

Figure 6.6 *(continued)*

(g)

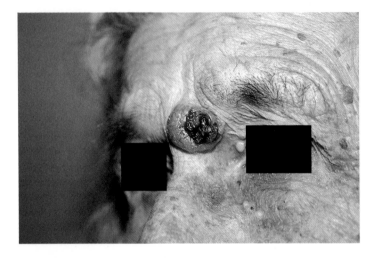

(h)

(i)

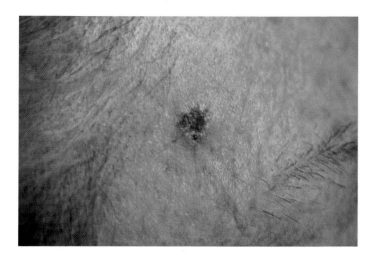

Figure 6.7

(a) Superficial BCC of temple.

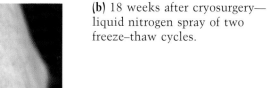

(b) 18 weeks after cryosurgery—liquid nitrogen spray of two freeze–thaw cycles.

freeze–thaw cycle that is needed to eradicate solid, cystic or ulcerated rodent ulcers.

Physicians embarking on cancer cryosurgery should start by treating tumours which might otherwise be treated by curettage and cautery or simple excision and primary closure (Figure 6.7). Until greater skill is acquired, it is best to avoid sites that have the higher recurrence rates

(e.g. inner canthus, nasolabial folds and periauricular lesions). For experienced cryosurgeons, the ear, eyelid and cartilaginous parts of the nose are relatively good sites for cryosurgery because cartilage necrosis is not likely with routine methods (Burge et al, 1984) and connective tissue damage and distorting scars are rare (Shepherd and Dawber, 1984) (Figure 6.8).

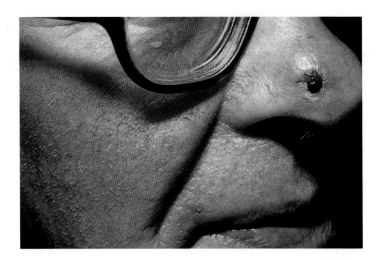

Figure 6.8

(a) Nasal BCC.

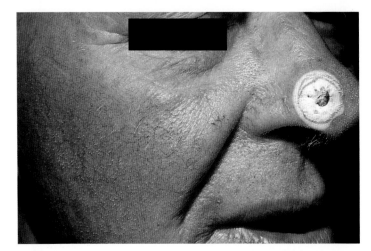

(b) During treatment.

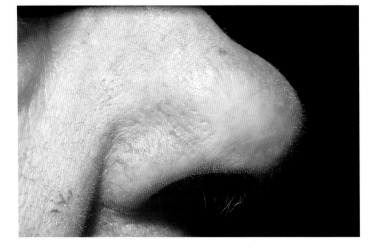

(c) 3 months post-therapy.

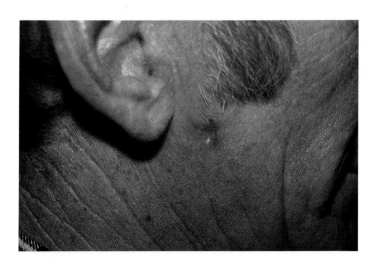

Figure 6.9

(a) Morphoeic BCC before treatment.

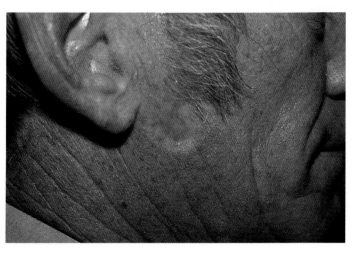

(b) After therapy by double 30 s freeze–thaw cycle, leaving some atrophy, hypopigmentation and loss of follicles. No recurrence at 5 years.

In treatment of a solid or cystic-type basal cell carcinoma, the lesion to be treated is first outlined with a marker pen leaving a 3 mm clinically clear margin. The complete area to be treated is then infiltrated by local anaesthetic. If the margins are not clear it is unwise for an inexperienced operator to continue (Figure 6.9).

In treatment of a well-circumscribed malignancy, the liquid nitrogen is applied as a spray either directly or through an open cone, of appropriate diameter, which is pressed firmly against the outlined lesion.

In treatment of a basal cell carcinoma, either of irregular outline or near a structure which might need protection (e.g. the eye), adhesive putty can be used to circumscribe the lesion together with a 3 mm margin. A double freeze–thaw cycle is then carried out to achieve subzero temperatures of at least

–40°C or to maintain the lateral ice line for 25–30 seconds with a minimum intervening thaw time of 5 minutes.

Basal cell carcinomas greater than 2 cm in diameter should be treated by dividing up the area into overlapping 2 cm circles and treating each circle separately by the spot-freeze technique, which has been previously described (Chapter 3).

If one has to deal with either a morphoeic, more invasive basal cell carcinoma or one with a poorly demarcated margin, then cryosurgery may not be the modality of choice. Many dermatologists would recommend wide excision or Mohs' surgery. If cryosurgery is used for any reason, then it is essential to include a 5–6 mm margin around the tumour.

Squamous cell carcinoma

Population studies and clinical research have suggested various aetiological factors in the development of this malignant tumour (Figure 6.10(a–h)). These include sun (ultraviolet radiation) exposure, polycyclic hydrocarbons, ageing, certain chronic skin diseases and the human papilloma virus; it is common in immunosuppressed individuals.

Squamous cell carcinoma arises on skin that is already damaged, most commonly as a result of exposure to ultraviolet radiation. The 'typical' patient is an elderly male and the most common sites are the face, neck, the back of the hand and the forcarm. The lesion usually presents as a firm, indurated, expanding nodule, not uncommonly on the site of a pre-existing actinic keratosis. The squamous cell carcinoma grows more rapidly than basal cell carcinoma. It grows laterally and vertically and may metastasize to local draining lymph nodes or distant sites.

Well-differentiated squamous cell carcinomas related to sun damage require two freeze–thaw cycles to avoid treatment failure or frequent recurrence (Kuflick and Gage, 1991) (Figures 6.11 and 6.12).

Unlike the basal cell lesion, the squamous carcinoma more often invades underlying tissue such as cartilage. If aggressive cryosurgery is used, a permanent structural defect may occur. Even though good cure rates can be obtained, cryosurgery is probably best avoided as a first-line treatment for lesions on the ear.

The clinical signs of squamous cell carcinoma in the early stages are less clear cut than those of basal cell carcinomas. Therefore diagnosis prior to treatment of a squamous cell carcinoma is essential. Because of this, very small lesions are better treated by excisional biopsy if primary closure is possible. Cryosurgery treatment for larger lesions involves a full double 30 second freeze–thaw cycle, using a cryospray cone of appropriate size, or simple cryospray using the spot-freeze technique, with or without an 'adhesive putty shield' (Figure 6.13).

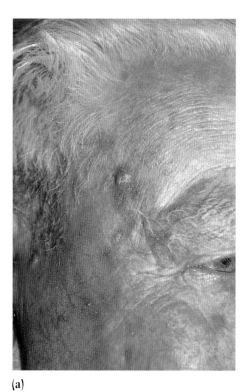

(a)

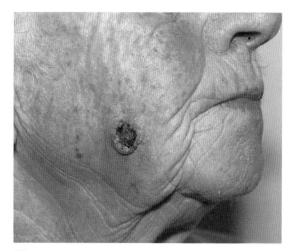

(b)

(c)

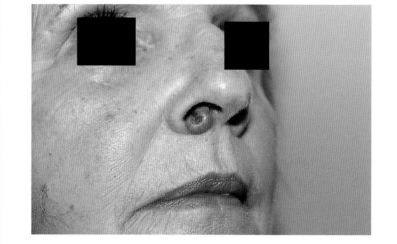

Figure 6.10

(a–h) Squamous cell carcinoma—
various morphological types.

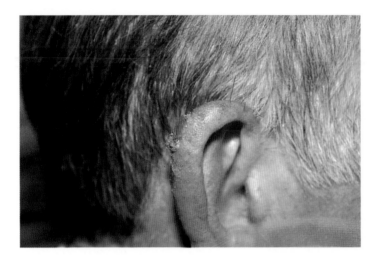

Figure 6.10 *(continued)*

(d)

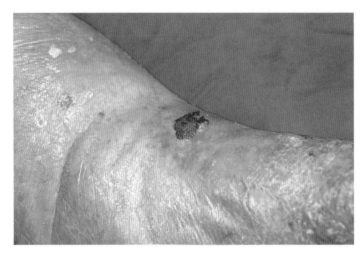

(e)

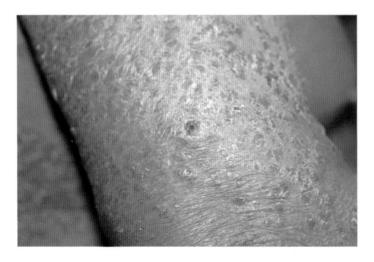

(f)

(g)

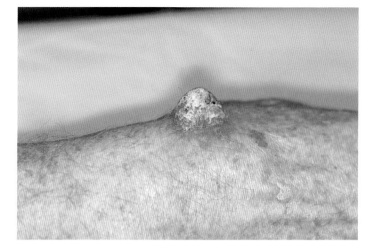

(h)

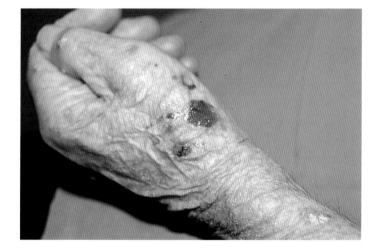

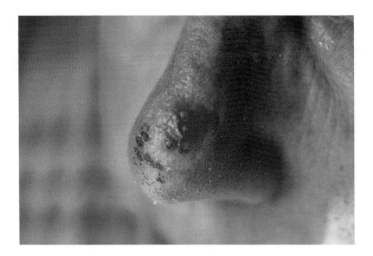

Figure 6.11

(a) SCC of tip of nose.

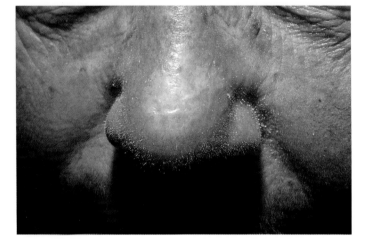

(b) Response to double freeze (30 s)–thaw cycle cryosurgery, liquid nitrogen spray.

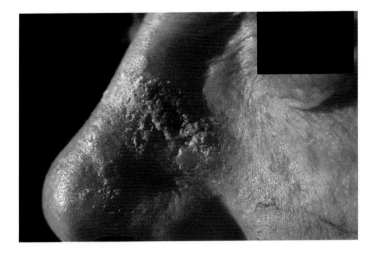

Figure 6.12
(a) SCC of bridge of nose.

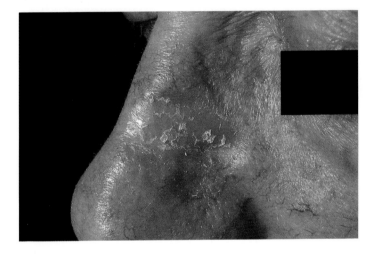

(b) Slight hyperpigmentation following cryosurgery (single 30 s freeze).

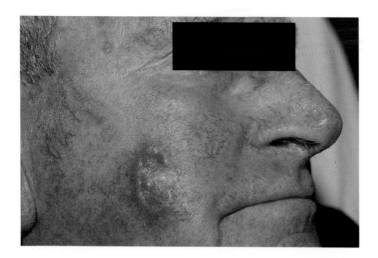

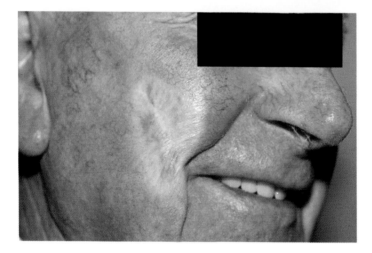

Figure 6.13

(a) Large SCC of cheek.

(b) 10 months after cryosurgery.

Lentigo maligna and lentigo maligna melanoma

Dermatologists have been using freezing techniques for lentigo maligna for many decades (Zacarian, 1982). Anecdotal reports have always appeared good. Dawber and Wilkinson (1979), published a series with long follow-up observations confirming the long-held view that aggressive cryosurgery gives satisfactory cure rates (Figure 6.14).

Bearing in mind the relatively large size of lentigo maligna, most frequently on the face in the elderly, the decision as to the choice of treatment depends on the general health of the patient and other circumstances such as ease of access and availability of treatment.

Where cryosurgery is the treatment of choice, a pre-treatment incisional edge or punch biopsy is essential. However, it is important to realise that the biopsy, even when taken from the most pigmented area, does not necessarily give the maximum depth of the lesion. Hence it is wise to use an aggressive cryosurgery regime (i.e. a double 30 second FTC) with a 3–5 mm lateral margin to ensure adequate depth and lateral spread of cryofreeze and cell death.

Despite what has been said in the previous paragraph, cryosurgery can have a palliative role in the treatment of malignant melanoma. Whilst cryobiological research confirms the sensitivity which normal melanocytes exhibit to cryofreeze, excisional surgery remains the correct treatment for malignant melanoma.

Studies are continuing on the use of cryosurgery for malignant melanoma. This must be considered experimental (Zacarian, 1991) and an area of obvious interest to all cryosurgeons (Figure 6.15).

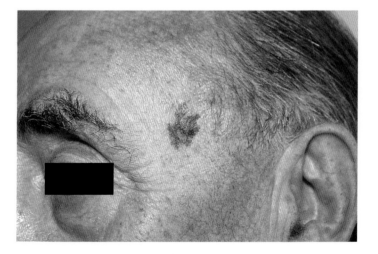

Figure 6.14

Lentigo maligna with recent changes in size and pigmentation.

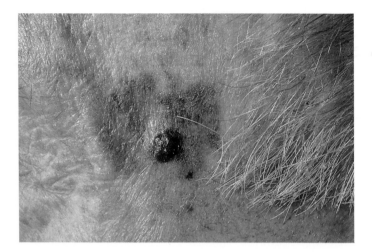

Figure 6.15

Invasive malignant lentigo with central nodule; **(a)** pretreatment.

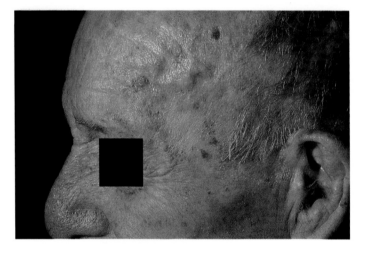

(b) 8 months following cryosurgery.

Palliation

Arnott (1851) showed the value of freezing temperatures applied to surface malignant lesions—decreasing the size of primary and secondary (often fungating) malignancies in the skin. Pain in such tumours was also often decreased and any chronic bacterial infections usually improved or were cured. In parts of the world where surgical facilities and irradiation are not available, such palliative methods are still useful. Liquid nitrogen is, however, a better 'killing' refrigerant than Arnott's salt–ice mixtures. Kuflick (1985) has shown that cryosurgery is still a useful therapy for many 'incurable' malignant skin lesions. Liquid nitrogen is so widely available around the world in hospitals, veterinary practices, biological units (mostly for tissue preservation) and industry, that it can be obtained even in developing countries (Figure 6.16).

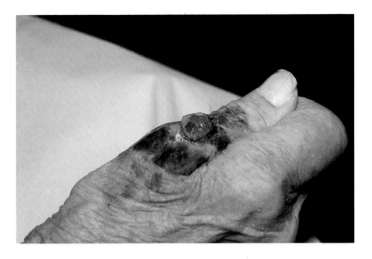

Figure 6.16

(a) Recurrent bleeding from a malignant melanoma in a 91-year-old, demented, house-bound patient—surgery not possible.

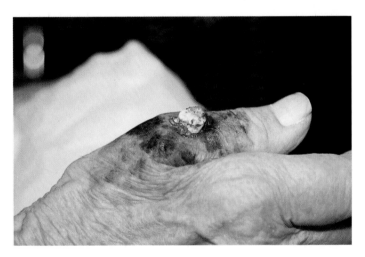

(b) Following first 30 s freeze–thaw cycle using liquid nitrogen cryocone—carried out as palliation.

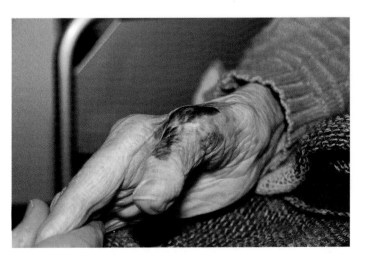

(c) 6 months following cryosurgery (good healing and symptom-free).

Recurrence and follow-up

As stated previously, failure of treatment following cryosurgcry is often due to poor technique. Recurrence rates, however, are higher in lesions greater than 3 cm in diameter. Ill-defined, more invasive, morphoeic basal cell carcinomas have a higher incidence of recurrence than superficial or solid basal cell carcinomas, and even squamous cell carcinomas (Kingston et al, 1988). Recurrences are also more common following treatment of rodent ulcers in certain areas of the face such as the periaural region, the inner canthus and the nasolabial fold. Some experts would consider excisional surgery a more appropriate modality of treatment for larger skin malignancies or those with higher risk of recurrence.

Tumour recurrences are best treated by a specialist with experience in skin cancer management. This might involve radiotherapy or wide excision with or without histological control of margins.

Studies have shown that most recurrences following cryosurgery are detected 12–18 months following treatment and certainly by 2 years (Holt, 1988, Kingston, 1988). Although good wound care following cryosurgery is essential, in most cases routine follow-up after wound healing has not been proven to be either necessary or cost-effective, provided that patients are instructed to report any problems at the treatment site or evidence of new skin lesions. The exceptions to this are patients with multiple solar keratoses or lesions at inaccessible sites, and patients who have had treatment of larger lesions or whose lesions were at the high-risk sites already mentioned. Routine follow-up of this group of patients at 12 months, 18 months, 2 years and then annually is sensible in order to pick up early malignancies or recurrences.

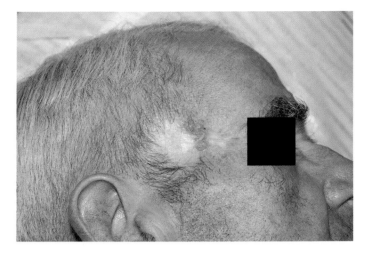

Figure 6.17

(a) Recurrence of a solid BCC of temple previously treated by cryosurgery.

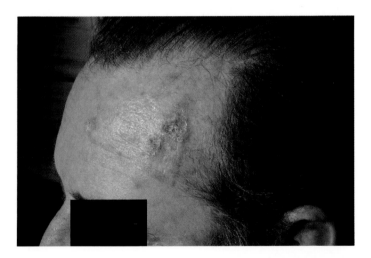

(b) Squamous cell carcinoma.

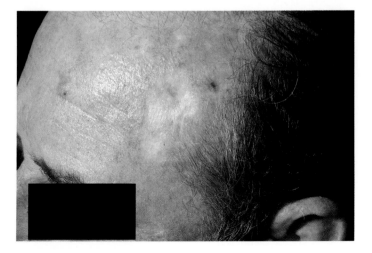

(c) early recurrence at 14 months following cryosurgery.

Advantages of cryosurgery

From what has been discussed in this and previous chapters, it is evident that cryosurgical equipment and skills could beneficially be available in all dermatology and surgical departments where there is outpatient treatment of skin tumours.

The advantages are:

- A low-risk outpatient procedure avoiding the need for hospitalization with its attendant inconvenience and cost;
- No need for general anaesthesia and only occasional local anaesthesia;
- A time-saving procedure which can be performed quickly and requires a minimum of outpatient visits;
- Multiple tumours can be treated at the same time;
- No need for strict asepsis (secondary infection is rare);
- Complications (e.g. postoperative bleeding from the surgical site) are rare;
- Cosmetic results are usually excellent;
- The cure rate is very high in properly selected cases.

The easily learned techniques and relatively low cost make cryosurgery suitable for use in primary health care as an extension of minor surgical procedure (Jackson, 1991). The additional advantages in such circumstances are improved services to the patient by:

- Reducing waiting time for appropriate treatment;
- Providing treatment in a familiar environment;
- Making better use of trained primary care doctors and nurses, with enhanced job satisfaction;
- Providing easy access for follow-up visits;
- Reducing hospital waiting lists;
- Providing a more cost-effective service.

Cryosurgery can be used with excellent results in the treatment of a wide variety of benign skin lesions and certain skin cancers. Its ease of use and relatively few side-effects make it a worthwhile modality for treatment of many patients in both hospital outpatient clinics and primary health care.

Table 6.4   Practical treatment schedules

Malignant lesions Lesion	Technique	Time (secs)	FTC	Margin	Sessions	Interval (weeks)	Response
BCC	OS or P	30	2	5 mm	1	—	92–99%
SCC	OS	30	2	5 mm	1	—	94–98%
Lentigo maligna melanoma	OS	30	2	5 mm	1	—	85–96%
Melanoma metastases – palliation	OS or P	30	2	5 mm	1	—	92% flat, healed and no clinical 'activity'
Kaposi's sarcoma							
AIDs related	OS	30	1	5 mm	1	—	84%
Non-AIDS	OS	30	2	5 mm	1	—	74–93%

OS = Open spray (times relate to spot freeze method—see script), P = probe.
These are 'average' freeze schedules.

Atlas of clinical practice

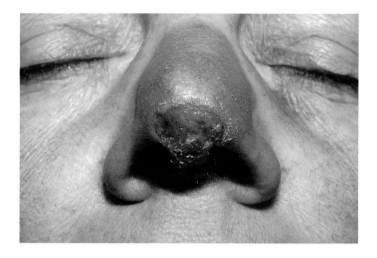

Figure 6.18

(a) Rodent ulcer of tip of nose.

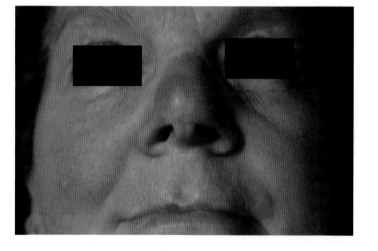

(b) Healthy recovery following cryosurgery—a single freeze–thaw cycle of liquid nitrogen spray.

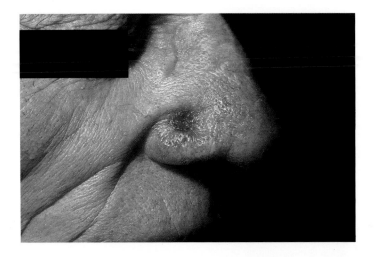

Figure 6.19

(a) Rodent ulcer of ala nasi.

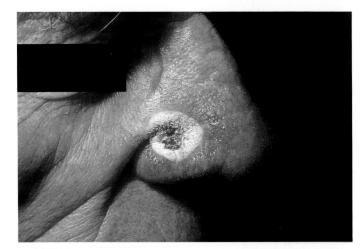

(b) Spot–freeze of lesion: $2 \times 30s$ freeze-thaw cycles, liquid nitrogen spray.

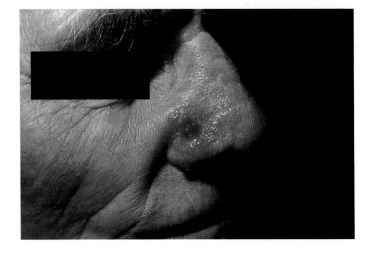

(c) Early reaction to cryofreeze—24 hours after treatment.

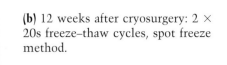

(**d**) Some hypopigmentation and loss of pilosebaceous units following treatment—4 months after treatment.

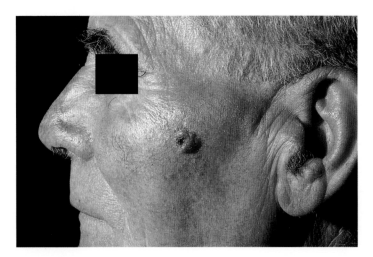

Figure 6.20

(**a**) Pigmented BCC.

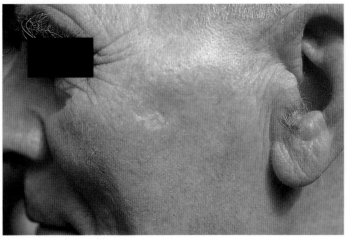

(**b**) 12 weeks after cryosurgery: 2 × 20s freeze–thaw cycles, spot freeze method.

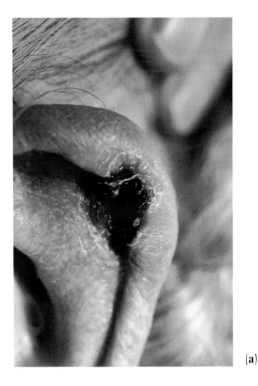

(a)

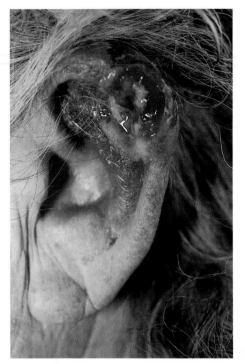

(b)

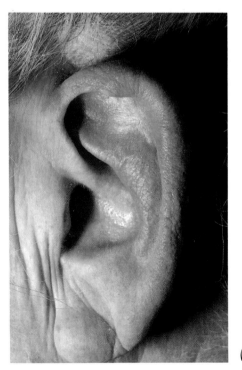

(c)

Figure 6.21

(a) Eroding BCC (rodent ulcer) of helix of ears;
(b) tissue reaction following vigorous cryosurgery;
(c) excellent resolution with no loss of cartilage.

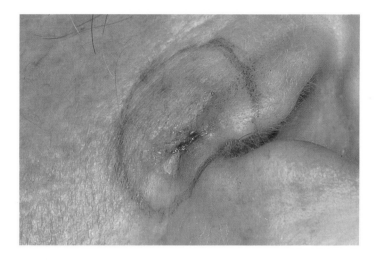

Figure 6.22

(a) Basal cell carcinoma pretragus lesion outlined with a good margin.

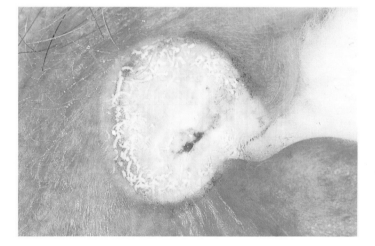

(b) External auditory meatus protected by cotton-wool bud and tumour treated by double freeze–thaw cycle.

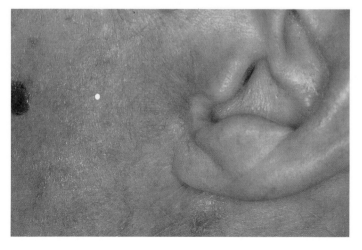

(c) Excellent outcome—15 weeks after treatment.

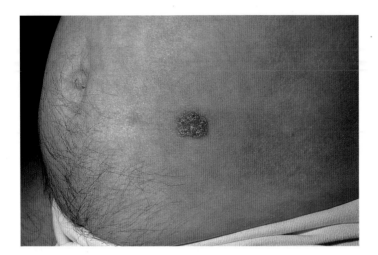

Figure 6.23

(a) Pigmented BCC of abdomen.

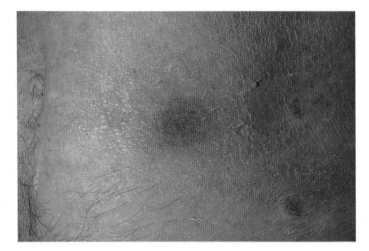

(b) Cryosurgery (one freeze–thaw cycle) resulting in some hyper-pigmentation—14 weeks after treatment.

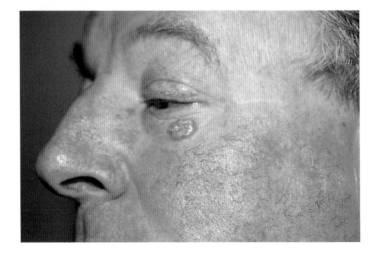

Figure 6.24

(a) Cystic BCC of lower eyelid:

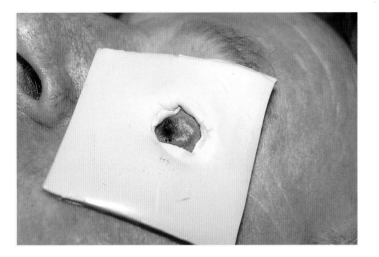

(b) Following curettage biopsy and with an adhesive putty shield in place.

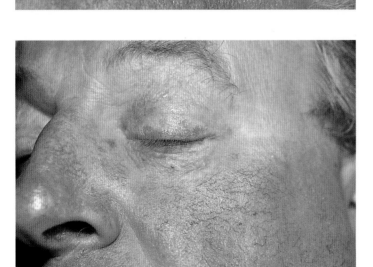

(c) Immediately after the first of two 25-second freeze-thaw cycles.

(d) 3 months after treatment.

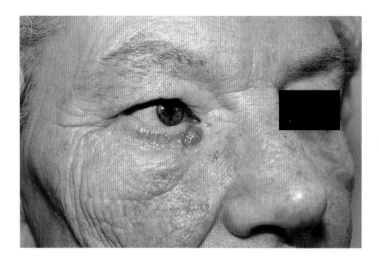

Figure 6.25

(a) BCC below lower eyelid.

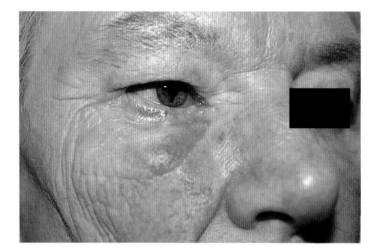

(b) 4 months following cryosurgery using cryoprobe technique – no loss of cartilage resulting.

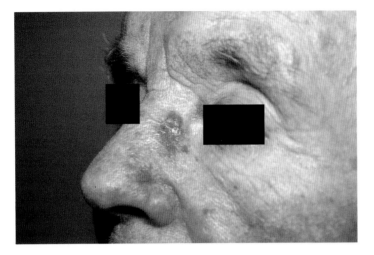

Figure 6.26

(a) Nasal BCC.

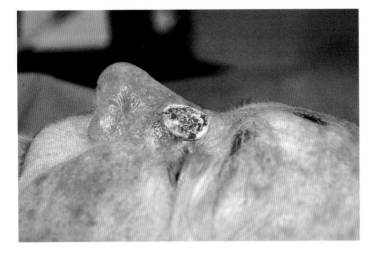

(b) Immediately following cyrosurgery.

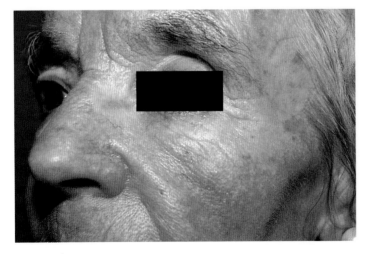

(c) 3 months after treatment.

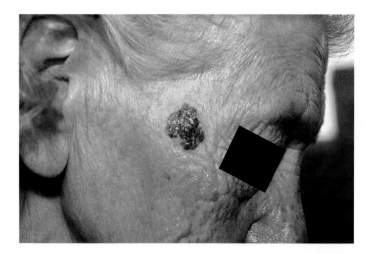

Figure 6.27

(a) Lentigo maligna in 80-year-old woman.

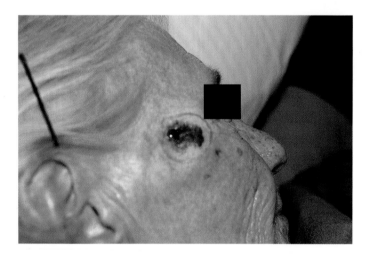

(b) Lesion outlined with clear margin and edge biopsy carried out.

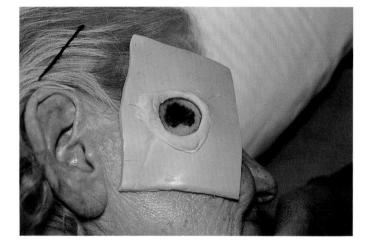

(c) Protective adhesive putty in place.

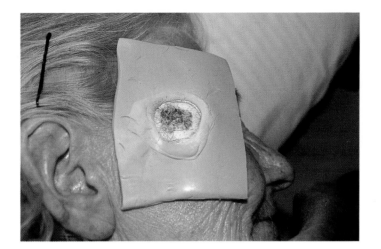

(**d**) Following 30 s cryofreeze.

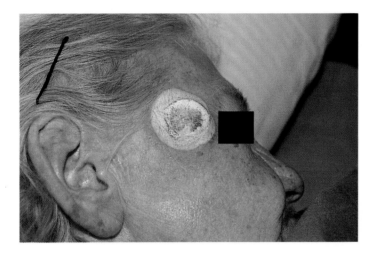

(**e**) Adhesive putty removed shortly after second 30 s freeze (note extent of icefield).

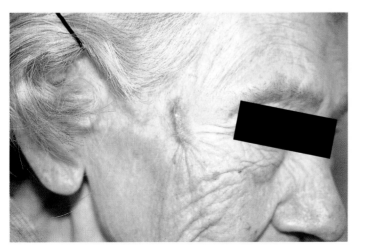

(**f**) Six months' review (hypertrophic scar subsequently flattened spontaneously).

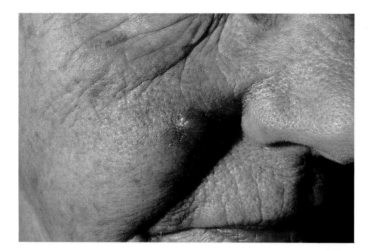

Figure 6.28

Lentigo maligna melanoma;
(a) early invasive melanoma.

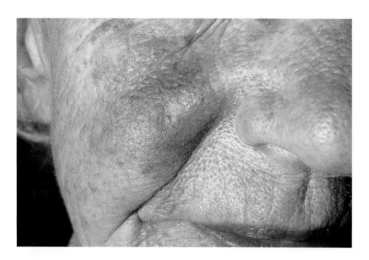

(b) 4 months following cryosurgery
(two freeze–thaw cycles).

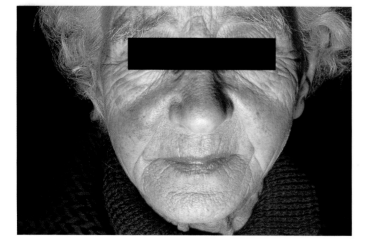

(c) 10 months following
cryosurgery.

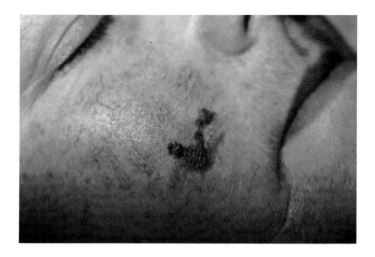

Figure 6.29

(a) Lentigo maligna (Hutchinson's melanotic freckle), an intraepidermal lesion, precryosurgery.

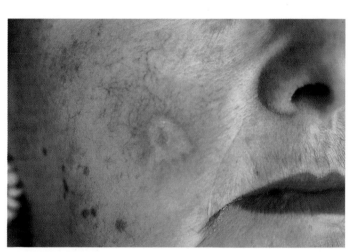

(b) 4 months postcryosurgery.

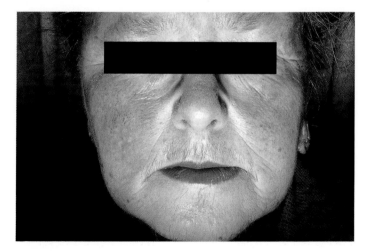

(c) 18 months following treatment.

Bibliography

Arnott J (1851), *On the treatment of cancer by the regulated application of an anaesthetic temperature* (London, J Churchill).

Burge S, Shepherd JP, Dawber RPR (1984), Effect of freezing the helix and rim or edge of the human and pig ear, *J Dermatol Surg Oncol* **10**:816.

Dawber RPR, Wilkinson JD (1979), Melanotic freckle of Hutchinson: treatment of macular and nodular phases, *Br J Dermatol* **101**:47.

Holt PJA (1988), Cryotherapy for skin cancer: results over a 5-year period using liquid nitrogen spray cryosurgery, *Br J Dermatol* **119**:231–240.

Jackson AD (1991), Treatment of skin cancers in general practice, *Br J Gen Pract* **41**:213.

Kingston TP, Hartley A, August PJ (1988), Cryotherapy for skin cancer, *Br J Dermatol* **119** (supp. 33).

Kuflick EG (1985), Cryosurgery for palliation, *J Dermatol Surg Oncol* **11**:867.

Kuflick EG, Gage AA (1991), The five-year cure rates achieved by cryosurgery for skin cancer, *J Am Acad Dermatol* **24**:1002–4.

Mallon E, Dawber RPR (1996), Cryosurgey in the treatment of basal cell carcinomas: assessment of one and two freeze–thaw cycle schedules, *Dermatol Surg* **22(10)**:854–862.

Nordin P, Larkö O, Stenquist B (1977), 5 year results of curettage-cryosurgery of selected large primary basal cell carcinomas of the nose: an alternative treatment in a geographical area unserved by MOHS surgery, *Br J Dermatol* **136(2)**:180–183.

Shepherd JP, Dawber RPR (1984), Wound healing and scarring after cryosurgery, *Cryobiology* **21**:157.

Sinclair R, Dawber RPR (1995), Cryosurgery of malignant and premalignant diseases of the skin: a simple approach, *Australasian J Dermatol* **36**:135–142.

Torre D, Lubritz RR (1983), Special issue: Cryosurgery, *J Dermatol Surg Oncol* **9**:183.

Zacarian SA (1991), Cryosurgery in the treatment of skin cancer. ed Friedman RJ, Rigel DS, Kopf AW In *Cancer in the Skin*, (WB Saunders, Philadelphia) 451–65.

Zacarian SA (1982), Cryosurgical treatment of lentigo maligna, *Arch Dermatol* **118**: 89–92.

7 Complications and side-effects

It is evident from the previous chapters that cryosurgery is an important therapeutic modality in dermatological surgery. In trying to assess the circumstances in which this method is the treatment of choice for a particular lesion, it is clearly important to know and understand the potential side-effects and complications, since all methods of treatment have 'unwanted' changes; cryosurgery is no exception to this general rule.

Many of the effects of the freezing methods employed in clinical practice produce inflammatory changes that are probably important for successful treatment—therefore morbidity, side-effects, and complications cannot always be treated as separate entities in cryosurgery, as will be seen with many of the changes to be described. Specific complications will depend largely on the regimen employed and on the site, pathology and size of the lesion to be treated; most of these are described in other sections. In this chapter, therefore, only the general complications, morbidity, side-effects and contraindications will be considered (Dawber, 1990).

Table 7.1 shows a list of the more well-known complications and side-effects. We will consider some of the more common effects listed since anyone new to cryosurgery should have detailed knowledge of these in order to explain to patients the most likely events prior to healing.

Pain

All patients will feel some degree of discomfort when local anaesthesia is not used. The subjectivity of pain means that this varies from patient to patient; even multiple, prolonged freeze–thaw cycle methods cause but little pain in some individuals. However, a few generalizations are possible: even the shortest, cotton-wool bud freeze gives a perceptible sensation of 'hot' or 'burning'. Tissue-penetrating regimens and those methods giving rapid lowering of temperature and ice formation often give discomfort within seconds of their commencement (e.g. liquid nitrogen spray techniques), probably due to the preanaesthetic effects of freezing on cutaneous nerve endings. Pain during the thaw phase, particularly after 'tumour dose' methods, may last for many minutes and be profound and quite intense. Certain anatomical sites are more likely to produce pain—

Table 7.1   Some side-effects and complications of cryosurgery.

Immediate
 Pain
 Headache affecting forehead, temples and scalp
 Insufflation of subcutaneous tissue
 Haemorrhage
 Oedema
 Syncope
 Blister formation
Delayed
 Postoperative infection and febrile reaction
 Haemorrhage
 Granulation tissue formation
 Pseudoepitheliomatous hyperplasia
Prolonged – usually temporary
 Hyperpigmentation
 Milia
 Hypertrophic scars
 Nerve/nerve-ending damage
 Bone necrosis and arthralgia – mainly terminal
   phalanx of interphalangeal joints
Prolonged – usually permanent
 Hypopigmentation
 Ectropion and notching of eyelids
 Notching and atrophy of tumours overlying
   cartilage
 Tenting or notching of the vermilion border of
   the lip
 Atrophy
 Hair and hair follicle loss

particularly fingers, pulp and periungual area, helix and concha of the ear, lips, temples and the scalp. Even though pain of the above type is usually transient, a throbbing sensation after digital freezing may persist for 1–2 hours.

These factors sometimes make the choice of whether or not to use local anaesthetic difficult. In general, single-freeze schedules used for benign or preneoplastic skin lesions will not require local anaesthesia—this may also be the case with superficial malignant lesions. If time is available, or if the patient needs to return for further treatment, EMLA cream, applied up to 2 hours before cryosurgery may significantly minimise pain. Headache, often migraine-like, is not uncommon with freezing of lesions on the forehead, temples and scalp—this is usually transient but occasionally lasts for many hours; headache is not always directly related to the site of freezing.

Nitrogen gas tissue insufflation

Nitrous gas tissue insufflation is extremely rare and is most likely to occur with open spray liquid nitrogen techniques carried out immediately after biopsy, particularly around the orbit; it can be avoided by starting with only gentle spraying directed at an angle, or by using pressure rings or cones. In 25 years of cryosurgery experience, the authors have never seen this complication.

Oedema

Oedema occurs to some degree with every patient—a product of the acute inflammation and 'leaky' capillaries—the amount of oedema relating directly to the severity of the regimen carried out. Pronounced idiosyncratic oedema occasionally occurs even from short freeze schedules. The severest oedema is typically seen in lax skin sites—eyelids, lips, labia minora (less common in labia majora), foreskin (Figures 7.1, 7.2).

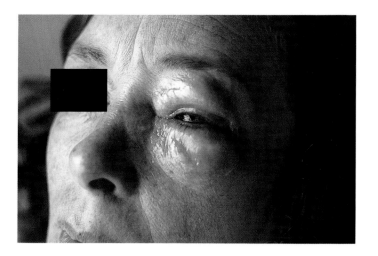

Figure 7.1

Oedema of the eyelids after treatment of xanthelasma of upper and lower lids with liquid nitrogen spray—probe methods are less likely to cause this degree of swelling. Swelling began within 2 hours of treatment and remitted within 2 days.

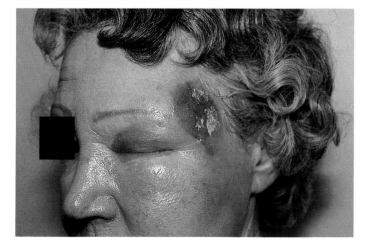
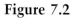

Figure 7.2

Oedema of the periorbital tissue may occur following aggressive freezing of lesions on the temple, as here, and the forehead.

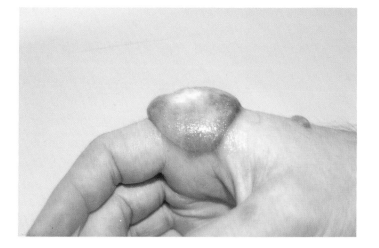

Figure 7.3

Haemorrhagic blister 6 hours after treatment of a common wart which can be seen surmounting the roof of the blister. Such blisters are only rarely painful and heal without scarring.

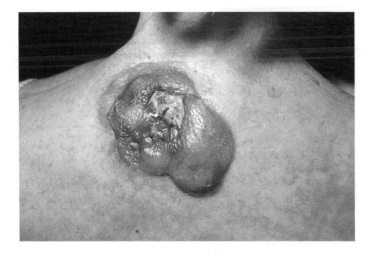

Figure 7.4

Haemorrhagic blister and necrosis 3 days after aggressive treatment of a large basal cell carcinoma. This degree of inflammatory reaction can be minimized by clobetasol propionate cream or a single dose of prednisolone 30 mg 2–3 hours before treatment.

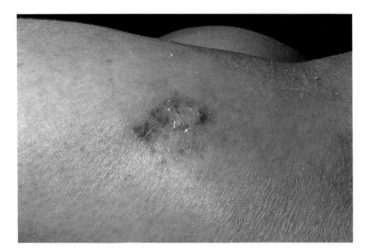

Figure 7.5

A large haemorrhagic bulla followed the treatment of Bowens Disease on the leg. This has healed remarkably well with a little residual haemosiderin staining.

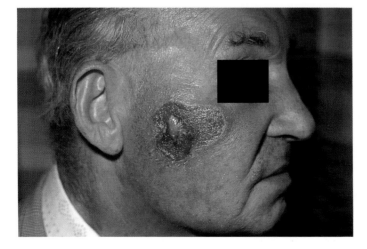

Figure 7.6

'Vascular' necrosis 6 days after two freeze–thaw cycle treatments for a 2 cm diameter basal cell carcinoma. Healing tissue remains undamaged and promotes re-epithelialization.

Whilst oedema equates with dermal and subcutaneous swelling, blister formation relates to the dermoepidermal split (see Figure 2.12) produced by the freeze schedules most commonly used in clinical practice (Figures 7.3, 7.4). Associated epidermal cell death may lead to 'weeping' erosions for several days. If sufficient capillary and venular damage occurs then haemorrhagic bullae may develop within 12–24 hours. Such blisters are often painless, presumably because of the temporary peripheral nerve ending damage; also they heal rapidly without scarring (Figure 7.5).

Haemorrhage and vascular necrosis

Within 4–7 days of aggressive cryosurgery, mainly tumour schedules, it is not uncommon for the treated field to become cyanosed with subsequent necrosis ('venous' gangrene) and sloughing of the dead tissue (Figure 7.6). This is probably due to delayed thrombosis of capillaries and venules and may be an important and necessary part of tumour death and high cure rates (Figures 7.7, 7.8).

Haemorrhage, sometimes excessive, may occur with cryosurgery by several mechanisms. If a pedunculated or prominently papular lesion is manipulated during its solid ice phase, any ice cracks that appear may be associated with bleeding during the thaw—this is usually capillary/venous bleeding and is transient. If cryosurgery is preceded by biopsy or curettage (e.g. to 'debulk' tumours), then postfreezing bleeding may last many minutes; it is easily controlled by application of 70 per cent aluminium chloride solution, rarely needing electrocoagulation. The rarest and most dramatic form of haemorrhage is the delayed type, up to 14 days after treatment. This may relate to the delayed necrotic phase after treatment of a tumour that had already invaded large arterioles or a larger artery—arterial bleeding of this type may be profuse and dangerous and requires immediate pressure to minimize blood loss and early tying off of the affected vessel. The authors have experience of one patient who bled from a deep vulval artery 11 days after a single, liquid nitrogen spray, freeze–thaw cycle treatment for multicentric pigmented Bowen's disease; she required transfusion of 4 pints of blood.

Inhibition of inflammatory complications

Most of the complications described above are the results of various components of the acute or chronic inflammatory reactions caused by freezing. Many attempts have been made to minimize or abort these effects without compromising cure rates. Some authorities recommend cyproheptadine three times daily for a day before, and several days after cryosurgery to minimize oedema; swelling and blister formation may be lessened by using topical clobetasol propionate, or oral or parenteral steroids (bolus-dose or short-term use).

Sensory impairment

Some degree of paraesthesia, or less commonly anaesthesia, is common after freezing. Indeed, the fact that cold can produce numbness has been known for many centuries.

The analgesic effect of cryosurgery has proved effective in the palliative management of various inoperable tumours by direct application to the tumour, while others have used a cryoprobe to produce analgesia in patients

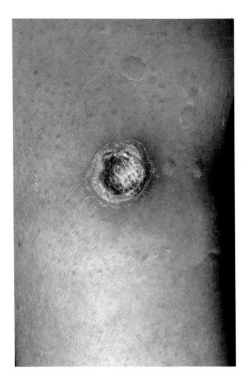

with intractable pain by blocking peripheral nerve function. These studies have also shown that, although all transmission is blocked in the frozen nerve, full recovery occurs after a variable period. This supports previous work directly freezing the sciatic nerve of rabbits with liquid nitrogen; in all cases nerve conduction was completely interrupted, but within 100 days, rheobase and chronaxie measurements confirmed full restoration of normal function. Thus, if a nerve trunk underlying a treated skin lesion is inadvertently damaged, complete recovery of distal sensory or motor function can be expected.

When skin, rather than peripheral nerves, is frozen it is well recognized that treatment of the affected area can be undertaken again several days, or weeks, later relatively painlessly. Pain after the initial freeze–thaw period of cryosurgery is also usually minimal. Although many studies have provided figures for the duration of pain relief after

Figure 7.7

Deep eschar formation after haemorrhagic and necrotic phase following treatment of Bowen's disease below the knee.

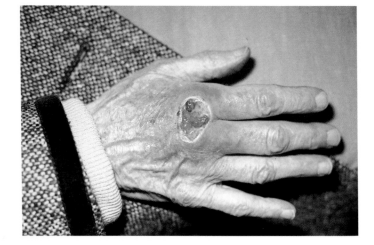

Figure 7.8

Erosion following two freeze–thaw cycles of liquid nitrogen spray for squamous carcinoma. Such lesions heal without the need for grafting, mainly because undamaged dermal connective tissue in the wound promotes healing without contractile scarring.

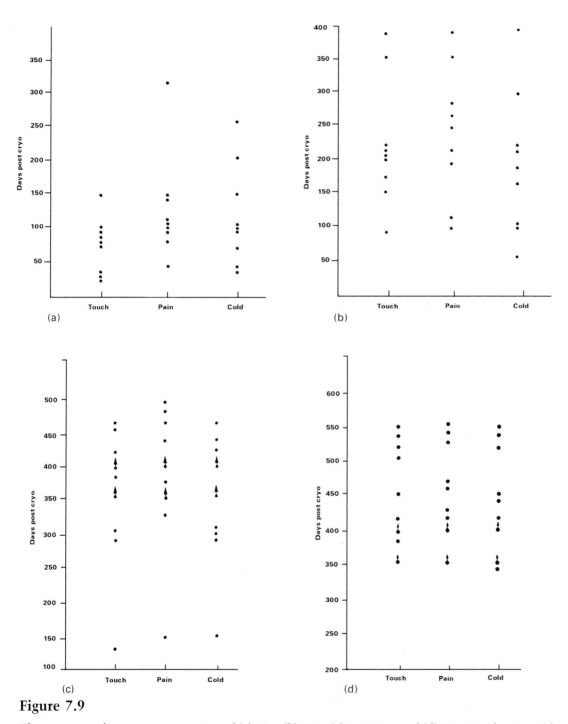

Figure 7.9

The response of cutaneous sensation of (a) 10 s, (b) 20 s, (c) 1 × 30 s, and (d) 2 × 30 s duration (after ice formation). The individual results represent the time at which that modality of sensation returned to normal.

cryosurgery to various peripheral nerves, there was, until recently, little information on the duration of sensory loss after cutaneous cryosurgery. Patients, however, require this information, particularly when a sensitive area such as the fingertip is to be rendered anaesthetic by freezing.

Subsequent work in Oxford (Sonnex et al, 1985) showed that appreciation of all three modalities of sensation tested (touch, pain and cold) was initially reduced in all subjects studied (Figures 7.9). The recovery took up to 1.5 years for the longest freeze. Compared with control skin, all treated areas sampled within the first few weeks of cryosurgery were found to have an absence of axons in the upper dermis and a noticeable reduction in the deeper dermis. The longer the freeze time the more pronounced were these changes. Even with the longest freeze time, however, Schwann cell and connective tissue pathways were present in normal numbers at all levels, with areas of Schwann cell proliferation. Apart from mild lymphocytic infiltration around a few of the neurovascular bundles, there was little evidence of inflammation and minimal fibroblastic activity. Dilatation of occasional superficial blood vessels was the only vascular change detected. Biopsy specimens taken at later stages contained increasing numbers of axons at all levels.

Faber et al (1987) carried out sensory testing by means of a graded bristle technique following treatment of 183 skin lesions in 169 patients—mild transient sensory loss was detected in 28 per cent of treated lesions; they noted that this did not appear to be influenced by the freezing technique used or the type of wound healing, but was site-dependent (the trunk and neck giving more prolonged impairment than the face; on the eyelid, however, sensory loss was not detected at all). It is, of course, these effects that may be the basis of the successful use of cryosurgery for pruritus vulvae and ani, the symptoms of lichen sclerosus et atrophicus, prurigo nodularis and lichen simplex (neurodermatitis).

Scarring

Hypertrophic or contractile scars are rare after therapeutic doses of cryosurgery (Shepherd and Dawber, 1984); if the former occur (Figures 7.10, 7.24, 7.25) they will require the same management as similar lesions produced by other modalities of treatment. It is generally stated that freezing does not induce scarring. From the work of Shepherd and Dawber, it has been shown that cryosurgical regimens that involve severe and prolonged freezing of the skin are quite capable of producing obvious scarring (Figure 7.11). Preservation of the fibrous network is the rule after treatment schedules used in clinical practice; this acts as a network around which cellular components regenerate. This process results in an often excellent cosmetic result, although dermal thinning may be a feature in the long term. Fibroblasts appear to be less susceptible to damage by freezing than epidermal cells. The possible protective nature of the blistering which accompanies healing deserves further in vivo study.

Paradoxically, early keloids (e.g. after ear-piercing) may be treatable by liquid nitrogen spray. Cartilage necrosis is extremely rare after freezing (Figure 7.12), therefore, ear, eyelid and nasal lesions give good cosmetic results after cryosurgery. It should be remembered that the only consistent exception to this dogma is cartilage already invaded by tumour—even if tumour cure is achieved, a cartilage defect may occur; this is more likely with squamous carcinoma than basal cell carcinoma (Figure 7.13).

Scarring in the general sense of permanent visual alteration in the skin appearance after treatment must include the effects on adventitious glands of the skin and hair follicles. Follow-up histology after tumour treatments consistently reveals loss of sweat, sebaceous and apocrine gland structures; indeed this information has led to cryosurgery being used in some centres to treat hidradenitis suppurativa, various components of acne vulgaris,

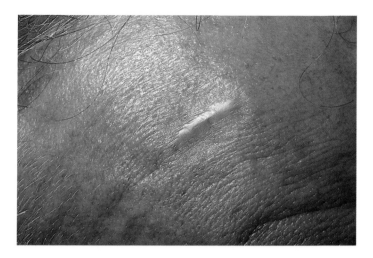

Figure 7.10

Linear hypertrophic scar 10 weeks after treatment (two freeze–thaw cycles) of a basal cell carcinoma—scarring of this type usually remits spontaneously within 6–9 months.

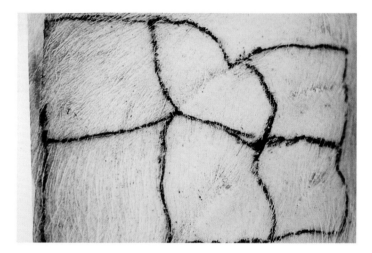

Figure 7.11

Skin on the flank of a pig: six 5 cm² areas were tattooed and treated with liquid nitrogen spray. The four squares to the right received doses in excess of those used in clinical practice and are distorted and contracted 3 months after freezing—compare the two left-hand square treated only with short 'therapeutic' range single freezes.

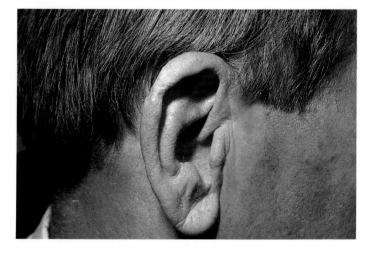

Figure 7.12

Ear—4 months after two freeze–thaw cycle therapy for basal cell carcinoma; only slight skin atrophy has occurred—no cartilage damage.

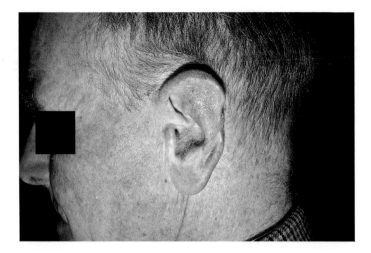

Figure 7.13

Ear cartilage loss—4 months after cryosurgery for squamous carcinoma which had evidently invaded the cartilage.

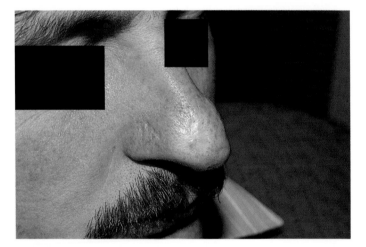

Figure 7.14

Loss of pilosebaceous pores and slight hypopigmentation following focal treatment of early rhinophyma.

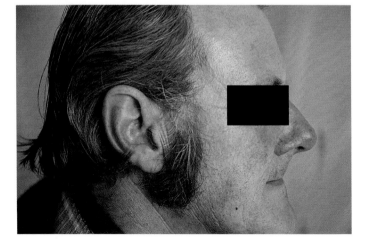

Figure 7.15

Hair follicle loss—permanent, following a single 10 s freeze of a flat seborrhoeic keratosis.

and axillary hyperhidrosis. Loss of the larger, normal, sebaceous pores after nasal and centrifacial skin treatments significantly alters the appearance of the skin and contributes greatly to the difficulty of cosmetically masking such blemishes (Figure 7.14). Hair follicle damage after other than the shortest freeze times is so consistent (Figure 7.15) that cryosurgery is generally only considered on sites such as the scalp and beard area for the treatment of small lesions; Burge and Dawber (1990) in Oxford have presented evidence to suggest that short freeze-times may sometimes cause 'resorption' and permanent loss of follicles without surrounding scarring, whilst 'tumour regimens' lead to overall dermal damage with associated follicular scarring (Figures 7.16, 7.17). The permanence of this loss suggests that the dermal papillae are irrevocably damaged by the freezing methods used in clinical practice.

Though dermal scarring is relatively rare after freezing, on non-hair bearing areas, epidermal atrophy may sometimes be seen (see Figures 7.21, 7.22).

Pigmentary changes

Postinflammatory hyperpigmentation is common after short treatments for benign lesions (Figure 7.18), particularly on below-knee skin; it may also develop in a halo distribution around a treated tumour site. If hypopigmentation or depigmentation occur they are usually permanent (Figure 7.19), even though nonfunctioning melanocytes may recolonize the white areas. As a result, patients should be cautioned about potential pigmentary problems (Figure 7.20). Cryosurgery is not usually appropriate for patients with dark skin types.

Contraindications

There are no absolute contraindications to cryosurgery; indeed, many of those listed in cryosurgical and dermatological surgery books simply imply that for many skin lesions, better cure rates can be obtained with other modes of treatment (e.g. morphoeic basal cell carcinoma), also certain sites and skin types lessen the usefulness of cryosurgery, mainly for cosmetic reasons (e.g. scalp and beard areas, negroid skin).

Many concurrent diseases may adversely affect the success rates and healing after cryosurgery. The authors entirely agree with Zacarian (1985) that the following diseases should in general preclude the use of cryosurgery—they are relative contraindications:

* Agammaglobulinaemia
* Blood dyscrasias of unknown origin
* Cold intolerance
* Cold urticaria
* Collagen and autoimmune disease
* Concurrent treatment with renal dialysis
* Concurrent treatment with immunosuppressive drugs (healing may be slower)
* Cryoglobulinaemia
* Cryofibrinogenaemia
* Multiple myeloma
* Platelet deficiency disease
* Pyoderma gangrenosum
* Raynaud's disease.

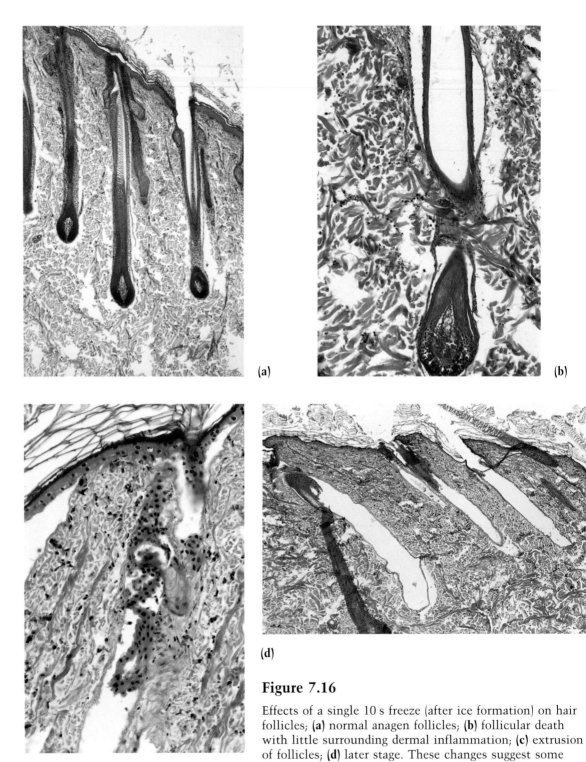

(a)

(b)

(c)

(d)

Figure 7.16

Effects of a single 10 s freeze (after ice formation) on hair follicles; (a) normal anagen follicles; (b) follicular death with little surrounding dermal inflammation; (c) extrusion of follicles; (d) later stage. These changes suggest some form of apoptotic resorption and dermal papillary loss.

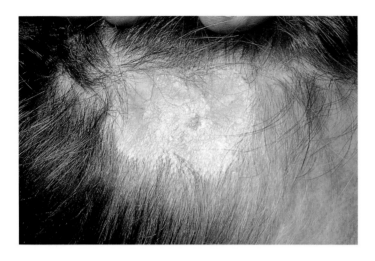

Figure 7.17

Scalp scarring following treatment of a basal cell carcinoma. In general cryosurgery is rarely a treatment of choice for scalp lesions.

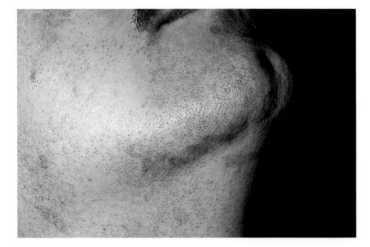

Figure 7.18

Patch (temporary) of hyperpigmentation after treatment of beard area warts.

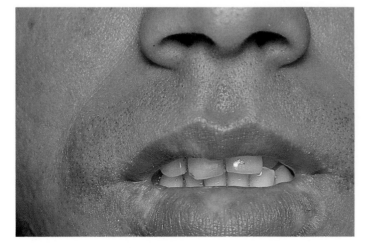

Figure 7.19

Hypopigmentation of lips in a dark skinned child after repeated cotton-wool bud liquid nitrogen for multiple flat (viral) warts.

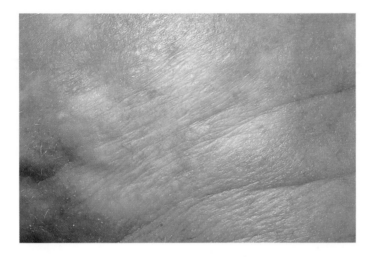

Figure 7.20

Hypopigmentation of the forehead following treatment of basal cell carcinoma—note the absence of contracting scar tissue (normal skin creases).

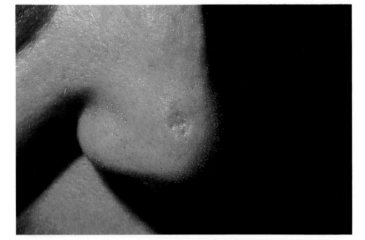

Figure 7.21

Slight depression at the tip of the nose following cryoprobe treatment of a spider naevus—mainly epidermal atrophy.

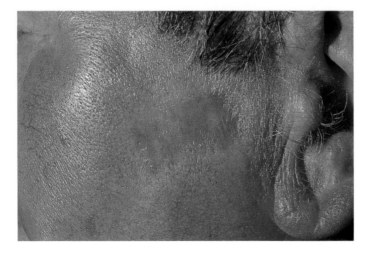

Figure 7.22

Epidermal thinning and telangiectasia—following cryospray treatment of a basal cell carcinoma.

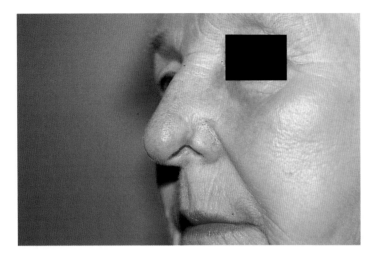

Figure 7.23

Nasal rim 'notching'—6 months after cryosurgery for SCC.

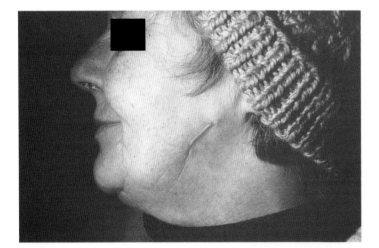

Figure 7.24

Linear hypertrophic scar 6 months after SCC treatment.

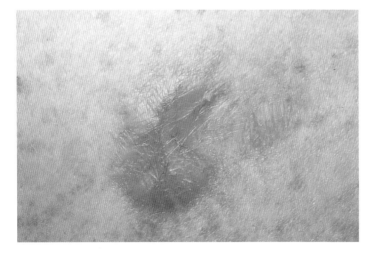

Figure 7.25

Hypertrophic scar—after BCCa treatment.

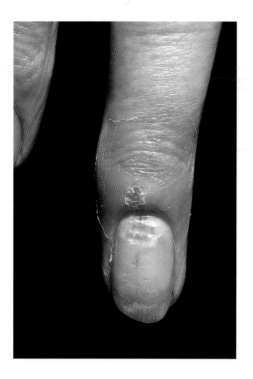

Figure 7.26

Transverse nail ridges/furrows after cryosurgery of myoid cyst.

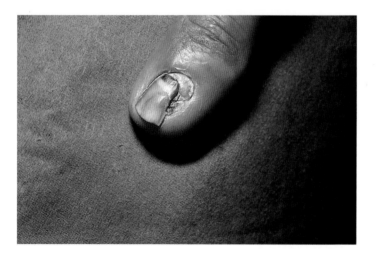

Figure 7.27

Nail shedding after cryosurgery for myxoid cyst.

Two of the most important contraindications are inexperience and the absence of an accurate diagnosis. Clinical experience is important but where there is any diagnostic uncertainty, a biopsy is essential. Cryosurgery is a destructive treatment but in the hands of a properly trained practitioner, it can have enormous therapeutic value.

Bibliography

Burge SM, Dawber RPR (1990), Hair follicle destruction and regeneration in guinea pig skin after cutaneous freeze injury, *Cryobiology* **27**:153–163.

Dawber RPR (1990), Complications, contraindications and side-effects. In: *Advances in cryosurgery: Clinics in dermatology*, ed. Breitbart EW, Dachów-Siwiéc E (New York, Elsevier) Vol 8(1), pp 108–114.

Drake LA (1994), Guidelines of care for cryosurgery. *J Am Acad Dermatol* **31(4)**: 648–653.

Faber WR, Naffs B, Sillevis Smith JH (1987), Sensory loss following cryosurgery of skin lesions, *Br J Dermatol* **119**:343–347.

Shepherd JP, Dawber RPR (1984), Wound healing and scarring after cryosurgery, *Cryobiology* **21**:157–169.

Sonnex TS, Jones RL, Weddell AG, Dawber RPR (1985), Longterm effects of cryosurgery on cutaneous sensation, *Br Med J* **290**:188–190.

Zacarian S (1985), Complications, indications and contraindications in cryosurgery. In: *Cryosurgery for skin cancer and cutaneous disorders*, ed. Zacarian SA (St Louis, Mosby Co) pp 283–297.

Index

Page numbers in *italic* refer to the illustrations.